129 easy ways to lose **disease and feel te**n

The

HONEY, GARLIC

and

VINEGAR MIRACLE

Ray Collins & Gareth Rees

The Honey, Garlic & Vinegar Miracle

129 easy ways to lose weight, beat disease and feel ten years younger

Ray Collins

© 2008 The Good Life Letter Ltd
Published 2008 by The Good Life Letter Ltd

The Good Life Letter Ltd
Emery House
Unit 7-9 Romsey Industrial Estate
Greatbridge Road
Romsey SO51 0AD
www.goodlifeletter.co.uk

Tel: 0845 675 1122

ISBN: 978-0-9557324-1-6

CONTENTS

PART FOUR
CONFESSIONS OF A FAT MAN: the honey, garlic and vinegar diet secret

PART FIVE
THE CHEF'S HEALTH KICK: 14 delicious honey, garlic and vinegar recipes

IMPORTANT NOTE

The publishers have carefully checked the contents of ***The Honey Garlic & Vinegar Miracle*** to ensure that it is as accurate as possible at the time of publication.

This book is here to show you the many historical and modern uses of honey, garlic and vinegar. Please be advised that the information in these pages is not necessarily representative of the views of health professionals and physicians. Do not treat this as a substitute for medical advice from qualified doctors.

In the case of any emergency, such as an accident, high fever or heart attack, please seek medical attention immediately. If you are worried that you may have a serious illness, please consult a medical professional before trying any of these home remedies.

If you are pregnant, we advise that you seek professional advice before you make any dietary changes.

Neither the author nor the publishers can accept legal responsibility for any problems that may occur when trying the ideas, tips and recipes in this book.

About the Author:
Health secrets of an information junkie

R ay Collins should get out more. His friends and family tell him this all the time. What kind of normal human being spends almost every waking hour locked his study, ploughing through websites, newspapers, magazines, journals and old books on a quest to rediscover lost natural health remedies?

For the past four years, this has been Ray's life as the principle writer for **The Good Life Letter**. Twice every week, without fail, this free email newsletter presents readers with ideas, tips and recipes scoured from every corner of the information universe. In simple, jargon-free language, he reveals little-known ways you can use natural food to help ward off disease, recover quickly from illness, lose weight and improve your energy and stamina.

In the past he's uncovered gems like these:

• How nuts could help you lose weight, fight depression and heart disease, and even lower your levels of bad cholesterol

- Why putting dill in your dinner could help relieve your irritable bowel syndrome

- The Japanese diet secret that could help lower the chance of developing prostate disease

- Why coffee could cure the morning blues and even boost your memory

- The amazing Chinese mineral lamp that many people believe can relieve the symptoms of joint and muscle pain, stress and skin conditions.

- How chilli peppers, cherries and peppermint could help relieve back pain

- The amazing chest-relief remedy discovered in an ancient Transylvanian mine

At first, **The Good Life Letter** was circulated around a handful of people who liked Ray's sense of humour and wanted to find out more about the many natural remedies that are cheaply available in the world around us.

Four years on, almost 30,000 people read **The Good Life Letter** every week. In return, they offer him their own tips, ideas and experiences. In this time, he's gathered an enormous amount of information on almost every ailment you can think of.

In 2007, I helped Ray publish **The Lemon Book**, revealing hundreds of ways you can use lemons to clean the home safely, treat minor ailments and solve everyday problems. Buoyed by its success, he immediately started work on this book you're reading now. This was great news for me, but annoying for his friends, who think he's turned into a crazed information junkie.

If you'd like to find out more about Ray's newsletter, go to his website at: **www.goodlifeletter.co.uk**. There you can read all his past issues for free.

Enjoy!

Gareth Rees
Editor

INTRODUCTION

Revealing the mysteries of honey, garlic and vinegar

A Miracle Cure –
Are You Kidding Me?

You could be forgiven for thinking this book is too good to be true. I mean, it's all about honey, garlic and vinegar. Basic food-stuffs you can find in your kitchen cupboard. And yet the book has the word 'miracle' in the title.

Can that be correct? Isn't the word 'miracle' a bit strong for what are, essentially, three ingredients of a decent salad dressing?

Miracles usually refer to amazing occurrences that science can't fully explain. But food? Have you ever seen a hunk of cheddar do the 'can-can', or watched your leftover carrots travel through time?

No, me neither.

But as you're about to discover, honey, garlic and vinegar have amazing properties that have mystified people throughout history. Their super-healing qualities have been well documented since ancient Egyptians engraved them into their temples and tombs.

I don't blame you for being sceptical. Like you, I get a little weary of opening the newspaper every morning to discover yet another 'superfood' has been discovered in some jungle somewhere, that it will blast away cancer and other diseases like a righteous hurricane, and that it will now be sold for £29.99 a bottle in the local supermarket.

I'm also cynical about food fads and diet crazes that may sell plenty of magazines and books, but cost ordinary people stupid amounts of money and never help you lose weight or feel any better.

But by the end of **The Honey, Garlic and Vinegar Miracle**, I think you'll understand why my title is no exaggeration.

Saving lives, from the Babylonian era to the First World War

As you're about to see, honey, garlic and vinegar have been used as health remedies throughout the history of civilisation. At certain points, they really were seen as miraculous gifts from nature. All three were known in ancient Babylonian times, discovered in the tombs of the Pharaohs, and even worshipped as gods.

They were dished out as skin treatments and cold remedies to the patients of Hippocrates, the father of modern medicine, while the ancient Romans and their Carthaginian enemies used them to fight infection, heal wounds, and even *smash through mountains*. (I'm not making that last one up, I swear. Just wait until you get to PART THREE and all will be revealed.)

In the Middle Ages, all three together were legendary protectors against the plague. In the 18th and 19th centuries they helped the European aristocracy stay perfumed, beautified and youthful. And on the battlefields of the American Civil War and First World War, they were essential antibiotics and antiseptics for the medic's kit.

If not *miraculous*, these achievements are at least wondrous, or phenomenal. And when you read on, you'll see that I'm only scratching the surface here. Wait until you hear about their effects on weight loss, blood pressure, asthma, stomach pain, headaches, tiredness, burns and fungal infections.

So forget what you *think* you know about these three items, which are probably sitting somewhere in your kitchen right now, lonely and underused. This book will be full of surprises.

Secrets of English queens, French grave robbers and Arab sexologists

You'll discover why bees are struggling with mobile phones, why dieters love honey, and why men in China have less chance of prostate cancer.

Weird? Perhaps. But there's more.

You'll also witness a terrifying battle between sharks, vampires and Triffids... read the dastardly tale of the French grave robbers who unearthed a life-saving secret during the Plague... go for a natural hair treatment with an English queen... get advice on impotency from an old Arab sex manual... and learn how a fat man in Vietnam lost weight without all the hunger, pain and rabbit food.

Best of all, when you eventually put this book down, you'll have a clutch of simple, inexpensive home remedies you can apply to almost any minor health problem. Instead of rushing to your chemists to splash out on the latest potion or lotion, you'll stop and think:

"Is there a natural alternative? Can I treat myself without all the artificial gunk and side effects? Can I do this without lining the pockets of a greedy pharmaceutical corporation?"

In which case, **The Honey, Garlic and Vinegar Miracle** will be an inspiration for you. In these pages, you'll discover:

- How to quickly knock up a cough medicine that's just as effective as the pricy stuff in the shops

- The amazing natural combination that could help you control your weight – drink this cocktail every morning and kick the food cravings

- How to reduce the appearance of wrinkles with honey and a cabbage

- A brilliant boost for your love life – the BBC's amazing 'discovery' about garlic and male impotence (the Chinese knew about this many centuries ago!)

- The Hippocratic solution for eczema – now you can relieve itching with a homemade recipe straight from your fridge

- How to make your own Vick's-style inhaler for a stuffy nose

- A dressing that controls blood sugar! Why pouring this simple mixture on every meal could help diabetics

- A ten-second remedy for bad breath

- What you *must* take the minute anyone in your office, workplace or home picks up a stomach or cold bug

- An easy way to blitz spots. This home-made remedy will blow all those expensive artificial creams out of the water

- An apple drink that could relieve heartburn

- An inexpensive and soothing athlete's foot treatment – this works wonders for any fungal infection at all

- Allergy sufferers! Here are twelve ways to clean your home without resorting to expensive products packed with chemical irritants

- Sleepless nights? This drug-free bedside syrup could get you back to the land of nod in a jiffy

It's all in this book, along with plenty more revelations. If you're trying to lose weight, stave off infections, protect yourself from allergies, keep yourself healthy and active, feel younger and fitter into old age, then there's something for you here.

My hope is that I can to provide you with an entertaining source of tips and ideas you can try at home, simply by opening a cupboard in your kitchen and reaching inside for one of these incredible ingredients.

Of course, there will always be those who dislike the idea of you turning to home remedies...

Why mainstream sceptics will hate you reading this

A lot of people will sniff at these ideas. Many sceptics can't stand it when I celebrate the largely ignored benefits of everyday foods, as if it's a crime against science.

You may even have to hide this book under a magazine on your coffee table when people visit. If a grizzled cynic sees it, he'll claim it's all part of this 'complementary medicine' craze. He may even say that what I'm offering you here is 'alternative medicine'.

Of course, it's not.

What's 'alternative' about honey, garlic and vinegar, three common natural antibiotics and antiseptics that have been used across the planet for over 5,000 years?

I'm not claiming that these natural remedies are a replacement for modern medicine. But it's your right to have access to this kind of information. And if just one of these tips helps you overcome an annoying health problem, it's worth the read.

Imagine if one of these foods – garlic, honey, or vinegar – didn't exist, and you suddenly invented it in a laboratory today. You'd have scientists and pharmaceutical giants scrambling over each other to get hold of your secret, patent it, and use it in their products.

They'd call it a 'scientific breakthrough' and make millions from it.

Unfortunately for the corporations, these natural resources are cheap, plentiful, and belong to *anybody*. You can't patent them. You can't own them. You can't stop anyone trying them out. And if you, a grown adult, wish to look into their beneficial properties, you shouldn't be mocked for it. Nor should this information be hidden or suppressed.

If the pharmaceutical giants and their private army of scientists have their way, a very unappetising scenario is possible...

A world without natural medicines?

Imagine a world where natural supplements are outlawed...

...Where health food stores are stripped of all their products and banned from selling anything stronger than a cup of water...

...Where naturopaths are forbidden to practise their craft, or fined when they try to pass on their knowledge...

...Where people with cancer, heart disease and Alzheimer's aren't allowed to seek out alternative remedies to ease their pain...

...Where they aren't deemed responsible or intelligent enough to look for their solutions to their disease, however slight the chance of a cure...

...Where books that promote natural remedies are bulldozed into large piles and burned.

It sounds like science fiction, but it's in the realms of possibility. The seeds are already being sown across the Atlantic. In the USA, the Food and Drug Administration (FDA) has been launching a quiet attack on all who practise, preach and supply information about natural medicine.

A document called the *'Draft Guidance for Industry on Complementary and Alternative Medicine Products and Their Regulation by the Food and Drug Administration'* has revealed plans to reclassify all vitamins, supplements, herbs – and even vegetable juices – as FDA-regulated drugs.

As regulated drugs, they would require FDA approval before anyone could use them or sell them as health products. This is not only an encroachment on personal freedom, it's a blatant attempt to force people away from the many natural options cheaply available to them in any local store. Options I'm going to show you in this book.

According to Mike Adams of *The Organics Consumer Association:*

"If the FDA gets its way, the United States will become a medical wasteland, dominated by corporate drug company interests, where the naturopaths are imprisoned and their products destroyed.... Simply selling dried broccoli sprouts as being 'good anti-cancer foods' may land you in prison, and running a vitamin shop could result in you being arrested for 'practising medicine'."*

Whatever you think of alternative medicine, this attack on natural food is going too far. These ideas smack of fear, arrogance and censorship.

The plant-life of this planet, with all its by-products, vitamins and minerals is our natural medicine chest. We should use it responsibly and with open minds.

It's your right to read a book like this and at least catch a glimpse of the sheer range of natural health remedies out there. Although when I say 'out there', I'm talking about ordinary items you find in your larder or fridge.

What is it that's so special about Honey, Garlic and Vinegar

For the past four years I've been a writer for **The Good Life Letter**. It's a weekly email service that provides insights into ways you can use food to live a healthier life, free of disease and common, niggling complaints. In the course of my research, I've been amazed by

*This quote first appeared in Natural News, published by Truth Publishing, Inc.

how many times honey, garlic and vinegar crop up.

Every week it seems that I get an email from a reader offering their own personal experience with these foods. (Along with the occasional email correcting my spelling, or asking me out on a date.)

Most strangely of all, one of the most popular remedies on my website involves a combination of *all three*. It's a very odd phenomenon: *where my readers have been using honey, garlic and vinegar to help shed the pounds* (you'll discover how and why in this book's thrilling conclusion.)

When I realised the connection between honey, garlic and vinegar, the idea for this book was born. I decided to collect all the recipes, remedies and secrets together. This way I could go to a wider audience with the exciting things my readers and I have discovered.

This is not intended to be a science book or a medical directory. Instead, I wanted to take people on a journey into the past to rediscover ideas and remedies that our forefathers and ancestors relied upon before the advent of modern medicine. So much anecdotal folk wisdom is being lost to the past, it seems a shame.

This is an attempt to dig it up, and bring some of it back to life.

To perform this miraculous act of resuscitation, I've looked everywhere, offline and online. I've sifted through long-forgotten recipe books, medical journals and alternative newsletters. I've read ancient legends, old wives' tales, and modern blogs. I've scoured internet forums for anecdotal stories and inspirational advice.

And a lot of ideas have come from my *Good Life Letter*, real people using these remedies in the real world.

In this book, I'll show you:

- A tasty morning drink that could kick-start your metabolism and help you control your weight

- The Louis Pasteur germ-killing remedy – how to quickly clean and cure nasty boils and wounds at home

- A natural chemical-free spray that wards off insects – you can even repel mosquitoes with your breath. (No more of that nasty DEET insect repellent!)

- The *legal*, energy-boosting drug of Ancient Greece. This could do wonders for your sex life

- Spoons of honey down at the pub! Could this be the craziest hangover 'cure' yet?

- A hiccup remedy that will amaze your friends and give them the impression you're an all-powerful healer

- The New Zealand 'wonder honey' that can treat indigestion, sores and leg ulcers.

- How to immediately ease the pain of a bee sting

- A homemade detox recipe that could clean and beautify your skin

All good, right? So here's how I reckon we should play this...

How to get the most out of this book

I've laid this book out so you can enjoy it in one go. Sit down with a cup of tea, flick through, and it should read like a very odd time-travel adventure story. That said, you may suddenly throw the book down, leap to your feet, and give one of the remedies a try.

Fair enough.

You can *also* use this as a dictionary of forgotten treatments for common ailments. I've separated the three ingredients into three parts of the book. The ailments are all listed alphabetically for you.

In the final part, I reveal how the three combined could help you lose weight, plus the diet secret I discovered from my personal experience. At the back there's an index to help you hunt for information on specific problems you might have.

Finally, you may be one of those people who keep weird and humorous books in your bathroom to read on the toilet. Don't worry, I'm one of them. And if this is where **The Honey, Garlic and Vinegar** Miracle ends up, I'll be honoured.

This book is supposed to make you chuckle. In my many years researching the health industry, I've realised that there's only one thing as po-faced and dogmatic as the mainstream medical establishment. And that's the *alternative* health establishment. One side is continually bruising the other, demanding censorship, refusing to listen. Both sides love to release confusing and scaremongering stories in the press.

The scientists demand that all mention of 'scandalous' therapies are wiped out. For example, in early 2008 they pushed the BBC to remove the entire complementary health section from their website, causing widespread outrage. Meanwhile, many alternative therapists refuse to address crucial issues when their practices are questioned, leading to distrust.

All of these ideological clashes are conducted with mono-browed seriousness.

The truth is, most people don't care about ideology. We just want to feel better. And most ordinary folk believe there's a middle way between the two. That you can use conventional medicine and natural remedies in combination, to great effect. And that you don't have to feel guilty or miserable for doing so.

Hopefully, I can bring a smile to your face, and strike a blow for common sense.

PART ONE

THE PHARAOH'S FAVOURITE
The amazing healing
power of honey

CHAPTER ONE

The story of a natural medicine under threat

It was a normal Saturday morning in the Collins household. While my wife cooked eggs in the midst of kiddie pandemonium, I was still in my pyjamas, scanning a clutch of morning newspapers for the latest health news. It's a tough job, but someone's got to do it.

As I reached the 'environment' section of *The Independent*, my gaze wandered past a headline that made me stop – go back – read it again – and again.

The headline asked: **"Are Mobile Phones Wiping Out Our Bees?"**

I thought to myself, "What? Even bees are using mobile phones these days! No wonder they're in trouble."

My head filled with images of bees trapped beneath their Nokias, attempting to text their Queen for help, thrashing their tiny legs on the keys.

Of course, this wasn't the story. It was far more serious, with potentially devastating implications.

The newspaper report was about a theory that radiation from mobile phones interferes with bees' navigation systems. German scientists believe that disorientated bees are failing to find their hives. Lost, and far from home, they die of exposure.

I've since seen some articles disputing the Germans' theory. (The conspiracy theorist in me wonders if these journalists are in the pay of big mobile phone companies.) But whatever the root cause of the problem, there's one thing that even the sceptics agree on: whole bee colonies are disappearing.

In a phenomenon known as 'Colony Collapse Disorder' a hive's entire population vanishes suddenly, almost overnight. Nobody knows exactly why, but it's happening across North America and much of Europe.

If this phenomenon comes to Britain, it will devastate our stricken farming industry. Bees pollinate millions of hectares of our fruit trees and crops, worth about £200 million each year. Another report in *The Telegraph* claimed that bees are worth up to £1 billion for the UK economy.

How bad could things get? Well, to give you an idea, Albert Einstein once said that if bees disappeared, "Man would have only four years of life left".

It's not only the crops that would suffer. Without bees, there's no honey. And without honey, we will miss out on one of the most important natural medicines available to us. The crime is that very few people know this. We think honey is a spread for toast, an alternative sweetener, or a flavouring for deserts. But it's so much more.

Ancient superfood

As you're about to discover, honey is one of nature's true 'super foods'. No, it's not some trendy modern health fad. This has *history*.

The Pharaohs of ancient Egypt worshipped the stuff. You can see evidence of beekeeping in the Sun Temple, built in 2400 BC. Priests offered it as a gift to their gods and even used it in their embalming fluid. Later, the ancient Greeks used honey as a medicine. The Romans loved to cook with it. Bees were also an important symbol of power for Napoleon Boneparte. His flag showed a line of bees in flight.

And no wonder humanity has been so fascinated.

It takes honey bees 50,000 air miles, visiting two million flowers, to make a mere 450 grams of honey. Their mission is to store up high-energy food for the queen and the workers over the winter. In all other species, the worker bees die off in winter, but not the honey bees, who instead feast on this complex and concentrated food.

And honey is *very* complex.

While 80% is natural sugar such as glucose and fructose, the rest is a heady cocktail of magnesium, potassium, calcium, sodium chlorine, sulphur, iron and phosphate, vitamins B1, B2, C, B6, B5 and B3, plus small amounts of iodine and zinc. Honey helps your body absorb calcium and magnesium from your food. And it provides a decent dose of antioxidants, which can help prevent disease.

This list of compounds and chemicals may mean nothing to you yet. But read on, and you'll see how they could help heal wounds, relieve cold symptoms, soothe skin conditions and much more.

CHAPTER 2

The health powers of honey revealed

What follows is an alphabetical list of the ailments which honey has been reported to help relieve or even cure in the past. You should also look these up in the index to see where vinegar and garlic could help, too.

Allergies

Hayfever is caused by inhaling pollen particles or when pollen gets into your eyes. The resulting allergic reaction can bring misery to your summer. It's not exactly easy to enjoy a barbeque when your head is radiating particles of snot.

The good news is that many sufferers believe that if you eat locally produced honey, you could help protect yourself from the annual nightmare.

The theory goes like this. Bees collect pollen from local plants to make their honey. This means that the resulting honey contains the same pollen that causes your hayfever. By eating this honey, you ingest elements of these plants, exposing you to the allergens in small doses, and helping you build up a natural immunity.

Some scientists dispute this, claiming that when you eat honey the pollen is destroyed by the digestive system. That said, I know a hayfever sufferer who eats local pollen and claims it has a positive effect on her hayfever. Or perhaps she *loves* the taste of dry spoonfuls of pollen, which I can't believe.

It's either that, or she's really a giant bee in human form, preparing to take over the world with her secret army of 'bee-people'.

Terrifying.

If you want to try the honey approach, make sure you eat a couple of spoons worth of locally produced honey every day in the run-up to hayfever season, and then throughout. At the end of the season, you can be the judge of whether it's helped you.

If people doubt you, simply laugh and pass them a tissue as their heads explode in a ball of sneeze.

Beauty treatment

I've included specific beauty treatments for scaly elbows, wrinkles and dry skin in this part of the book. You can look them up in their alphabetical order. But here's a very quick anti-bacterial beauty treatment you should try twice a week:

Wet your face with warm water. Now massage a tablespoon of honey onto your face. Wait a few minutes, then rinse.

Coughs and colds

"Honey is better at treating children's coughs than an ingredient used in many over-the-counter medicines", proclaimed *The Daily Telegraph* on December 4th 2007.

Almost immediately, a billion mothers, grandparents and ghosts of grandparents past all sighed, "Yes, we already *knew* that."

Honey is one of those 'old wives' remedies that is so obviously effective, most of us don't bother to investigate the science. It just *works*.

Scientists now believe that honey is effective in fighting coughs and colds because it contains natural antibiotics that can kill microbes. It also acts as an antioxidant, protecting you from cell damage.

The research trumpeted in Britain's mainstream press was carried out by Dr Ian Paul and his team from Pennsylvania State University. They found that children who took honey syrup had improved sleep, a reduction in coughing frequency, and a less bothersome cough. The results were as effective as dextromethorphan, the key ingredient in pricey, mass-produced cough syrups.

Honey, of course, is a much less expensive and more natural option. And it works on adults too. One of my regular **Good Life Letter** readers told me he had the beginnings of bronchitis in one side of his chest. He was told by his holistic practitioner, an ex-G.P, to go home to bed and to make a hot drink of thyme and single-source honey.

He took this mixture four times a day. By the second day, the pain in his chest was easier. By the fourth day he was about to go out walking, with no rattle in his chest.

Here's a version of his treatment that you can try:

> Soak an ounce of dried thyme in a cup of boiled water, covered, until cool. Strain, then mix the liquid with a cup of honey. Now put this into a glass jar and store it in the fridge (it keeps well for several months.) Take a teaspoon of this syrup several times a day as needed.

Or if you prefer a tasty drink instead, there's an alternative.

> Take some freshly chopped basil leaves, some crushed raw ginger and add to hot water. Now stir in a teaspoonful of honey and, once cool enough, drink slowly. This is good both for sore throats and colds.

My personal favourite of all the honey cough-and-cold remedies is the hot toddy:

> Squeeze the juice of a fresh lemon into a large mug. Add hot water. Stir in two teaspoons of honey. Breathe in the steam for a few minutes, inhaling through your nose. Now drink.

The added option that your doctor won't ever recommend, but really makes the hot toddy, is whisky.

Believe me, this one has been tried and tested. It's somewhat of a religion if you talk to people in Ireland and Scotland. Yes, it probably dehydrates you a bit. But as long as you've been drinking fluids all day, I don't see the problem.

Just keep it to a couple of shots per day – okay?

"Suuuuure, Ray", you slur, forgetting all about your illness, "I love you mate, sheriously...."

Cuts and burns

Back in ancient Egyptian times, honey was applied to wounds to heal them quickly. It was so important, it was embalmed with the Pharaohs. Because honey doesn't deteriorate over time they found remnants of it when they opened Tutankhamun's tomb in 1922.

I wouldn't recommend spreading ancient Egyptian honey on your toast. Before you take a bite you'll have moustachioed men poking their heads through your window, crying out: "Your breakfast is cursed, I tell you, CURSED!

Honey has stayed popular ever since the Egyptians. In the last two world wars poultices (heated cloths) with honey were still being used for treating cuts and burns. But somehow, as the 20th century 'progressed', we forgot all about this powerful natural remedy.

Instead we relied upon antibiotics. Too heavily, and for too many years, it turns out. Now antibiotics are beginning to fail us. Diseases that used to succumb to their wiles have mutated into forms that are now resistant to the usual treatments. Elderly people in hospital are now threatened by many potentially deadly bacteria, and antibiotics simply aren't protecting them.

In these worrying times, the ancient Egyptian staple is making a comeback.

"In hospitals today we are faced with germs which are resistant to almost all the current antibiotics," says Dr. Arne Simon of the University of Bonn. "As a result, the medical use of honey is becoming attractive again for the treatment of wounds."

Experts from his research team have discovered that even chronic wounds infected with multi-resistant bacteria can heal within a few weeks when honey is applied.

And it's not just Arne and his crew of boffins. Studies at Cardiff University have experimented on irradiated honey as an anti-bacterial weapon against superbugs like MRSA. In Russia, some hospitals which can't access modern drugs use honey with amazing success. And in September 2007 the *Los Angeles Times* reported that The Smith Gate Burn Clinic in Iraq is using honey to treat children's burns.

Honey heals so brilliantly thanks to a combination of factors. Its acidity is low enough to hinder the growth of bacteria. Honey can also absorb water from a wound, depriving bacteria of the moisture they need to thrive.

When honey is diluted by the fluids from a wound an enzyme is activated, which produces hydrogen peroxide. This is a great anti-bacterial agent. Honey has also been shown to reduce the inflammation and soothe the pain of deep wounds and burns.

So if you've cut yourself, or suffered a minor burn, here's what to do...

> Clean the wound area with a sterilised cotton wool or gauze. If it's a deep cut, use hydrogen peroxide to wash the surface. Apply honey on the cut as final dressing. Cover as you'd normally do with a cut. Repeat this process twice daily.

If the wound is very deep, or the burn severe, I don't need to tell you what to do, do I?

No, because I hope *you're already on your way to hospital!*

Diabetes

Honey is said to cause a lower rise in your blood sugar levels than refined sugar, which means it could be better option for diabetes sufferers. Honey is sweeter than granulated sugar, so you can substitute a smaller amount of honey for sugar. It also has lots of vital nutrients you don't get in refined sugar.

But there's a huge debate raging about whether honey really can act as a substitute. So please check with your doctor before messing around with your intake of sweeteners. This is this for your information only. If you, or anyone you know, suffer from diabetes, this will give you a possible option you can talk to a professional about.

Disease prevention

At the University of California, studies showed that test subjects who ate four to ten tablespoons of raw buckwheat honey every day had higher levels of antioxidants than those who didn't. Antioxidants are known to keep free radicals (the little blighters which damage our cells) firmly in check, helping you fight disease.

Some experts say honey contains as many antioxidants as apples or spinach. So a spoonful of honey in the morning could keep the doctor away better than an apple!

Try eating an apple coated in honey every day and you could

become utterly invincible. Doctors will run screaming down the street to stay away from you.

As further evidence to honey's powers, in 2004, the BBC reported that honey "could help fight cancer". A team of researchers from the University of Zagreb in Croatia claimed that a range of honey bee products stopped tumours growing or spreading in mice. Dr Nada Orrolic said, "Honey bee products could be a useful tool in the control of tumour growth."

As you'll understand, research is in its early stage. While there's no magic milkshake that I can prescribe to give yourself immunity against disease, taking a couple of spoonfuls of honey each morning may improve your body's ability to stave off serious illness.

It just goes to show how powerful honey is, that scientists across the world are still researching its potential.

Dry Skin

Honey is a natural 'humectant'. This means that it helps your skin retain its moisture. The Chinese have long used honey with ground orange seeds to keep their skin youthful. And today you can go for honey beauty treatments where honey and sesame oil is poured over you and massaged into your skin.

Madame du Barry, mistress to Louis XV, used honey as a facial mask. She's the one who was executed in the French Revolution after trying to smuggle jewels to England. Her last words to the executioner were, "Encore un moment, monsieur le bourreau, un petit moment".

This meant "Just one moment, executioner, just one moment more."

Why did she say this? I'd like to believe it was because she suddenly realised something really embarrassing – she still had on her honey face-pack!

Madame du Barry's life may have ended badly. But don't let that put you off trying a version of her face treatment:

> Beat an egg in a bowl. Add half a cup of coconut oil and half a cup of honey, still beating as you go. When it's thick and creamy, pour it into an upright tube, like the cardboard bit from inside a toilet roll, for example.

> It all sounds weird, I know. But stick the tube in the freezer overnight, then take it out the next day. Peel back the tube and rub the stick on your face, like a giant lip-balm. After 10 minutes, rinse it off.

Here's another tip:

> To keep your skin glowing like you bathe in the fountain of youth every morning, drink a warm glass of water with honey and lemon juice first thing in the morning. This will help you keep your system flushed of toxins.

Eczema

Hippocrates, the Greek physician and father of modern medicine, used honey for skin disorders. That said, at the time he didn't know that he was the father of modern medicine. If anything, he was the 'son of *ancient* medicine".

Anyway, many years on, science is waking up to old Hippocrates. According to reports in *Complementary Therapies in Medicine*, a mixture of honey, olive oil, and beeswax has been shown to relieve the symptoms associated with eczema and psoriasis.

Why? Well, the theory goes that the flavonoids in olive oil and honey help protect your cells. They also control levels of histamine, the substance involved in allergic reactions. These mix well with beeswax, which is another anti-inflammatory.

In the 2003 study, 80% of the participants with eczema had a significant improvement using the honey, olive oil and beeswax mixture prescribed to them.

This is great news for eczema sufferers, who are usually given over-the-counter lotions and prescription corticosteroid creams to relieve the itching. The trouble with 'corticosteroid' creams, however, is that they may cause thinning of the skin. Other critics say they can prolong the healing time of injured skin.

So honey, olive oil and beeswax could be an alternative solution. To make your own skin remedy mixture, here's what to do.

Mix two tablespoons of raw, or whole comb, honey (see Chapter Three for details) with two tablespoons of cold pressed olive oil. Now melt two tablespoons of beeswax in a pan. Then mix with the honey and olive oil mixture, stirring all the time.

Once it's all mixed nicely, put it in the fridge and try it later that day. It should keep for three months.

Fatigue

Each morning before your eat or drink anything, take a cup of nettle tea with a teaspoonful of honey. This has been known to treat intermittent constipation and chronic tiredness throughout the day.

Nettles can drastically lower your levels of blood sugar, which is why it's a good idea to add honey to the tea, especially if you're diabetic.

Fertility

The Scandinavian word for 'honeymoon' comes from an ancient Northern European custom where newlyweds drank a daily cup of honeyed wine every night for the first month of married life. Our Saxon ancestors thought it would keep people randy and fertile.

Is the ancient European theory so far-fetched?

Not according to Susan Fletcher of Norfolk bee products company, Apitherapy Foods UK. She says, "Put a woman who's struggling to conceive on bee pollen and you can pretty much guarantee a result within two to three months."

And indeed, studies have shown that bee pollen could be helpful in revitalising women's reproductive systems.

Supporters of bee pollen claim this is thanks to the natural hormonal substances in the bee pollen. It's packed with a high level of vitamins A, C, D, E and B. These help boost your immune system.

Companies like Holland and Barrett, Earthrise Foods, and Apitherapy Foods provide bee pollen products to the UK market. Have a search for them online, or in a local directory.

Gout

In 1628, a bad-tempered physician called William Harvey was having problems.

First off, nobody believed his theory that the heart acted like a pump, circulating blood round the body. No doubt the medical establishment of the time declared there was 'no official proof', so it couldn't *possibly* be true. He was probably seen as an alternative medicine quack and ridiculed by the local town crier.

Harvey's second problem was that he suffered agonising gout pains every night. It was so bad, he couldn't sleep. Instead, he'd clamber onto the roof of his house to do his thinking and theorising about heart pumps.

It was on the roof one night that he discovered a strange way to relieve his gout.

What he did was sit in his nightshirt with his legs in a bucket of cold water and keep them there until they were almost frozen. Then he'd run indoors to heat them next to the fire. Harvey, according to a report at the time, 'betook himself to his stove and so 'twas gone.'

In short, legend has it that he got rid of the pain with his own hot and cold treatment. This, however, is not my recommended remedy for gout. Instead, here's how some people believe honey can help:

> Mix four tablespoons of honey with a tablespoon of comfrey tincture. This is available online if you type "comfrey tincture buy" into a search engine like www.Google.co.uk.

> Next, heat the mixture in a 'double boiler'. A double boiler is also known as a 'bain marie'. This is a container placed

inside a larger pan of boiling water, so the liquid inside heats up very gently. This method of cooking is often used for cooking delicate dishes like custards or white sauces, or melting chocolate.

Once warm, dab this mixture onto a cloth and apply it to the painful joint. Leave it overnight. Repeat this for several weeks.

You should also try some nettle tea with two teaspoons of honey. This helps your kidneys and joints get rid of the uric acid that causes gout. The honey is important because nettles can lower your blood sugar levels quite drastically (see the section on 'Fatigue'.)

A final note about William Harvey: my spoilsport editor tells me that modern doctors now believe that he wasn't suffering from gout at all. Instead it was something called erythromelalgia (also known as Weir Mitchell's disease).

But I like the story, so I'm keeping it in this book. Sorry, Mr Editor.

Hair conditioner

You don't have to spend a fortune on fancy hair conditioners. Instead, you can follow Queen Anne's 'ye olde' recipe from the early 18th century.

This involves adding 100 grams of honey to 50 grams of olive oil and mixing. You then use it on your hair like ordinary conditioner, except you need to leave it for fifteen minutes before rinsing.

There you go. You look like you just stepped out of a salon. Well, first out of a TARDIS into an 18th century salon, *then* out of the salon. Hey, it's because you're worth it.

By the way, Anne died of suppressed gout, a natural remedy for which can be found in a previous entry. If only she'd owned a copy of **The Honey, Garlic and Vinegar Miracle**.

Hangovers

If you're out at a party, or just come in after a night on the tiles, baffle your friends by swallowing a teaspoon of honey every half hour until you hit the sack. The honey will keep your blood-sugar levels up.

My tip is to keep a small pot of it in your pocket. I realise that you don't believe I've ever gone out with a tiny pot of honey in my pocket. But this is what an obsessive I am. I try everything at least once.

Many drinkers swear that honey helps you fight nausea, headaches and indigestion. So don't worry what you look like if someone catches you having a spoonful. Just imagine how the other person's going to feel in the morning.

If you're drunk, and *they're* drunk too, there's an easy way to shut them up. Slap them on the back and say, "It's protection from the evil bee people" (see 'Allergies' for details).

Even the next day, it's honey to the rescue. The theory goes that the fructose in honey can help your liver break down the alcohol you've guzzled the night before.

According to the National Headache Foundation, honey on a cracker or piece of toast after drinking may prevent that 'near death' hangover. Dr. Merle Diamond, associate director of the Diamond Headache Clinic in Chicago, claims that the fructose in honey competes for the metabolism of alcohol. This means you don't get a sudden drop in alcohol levels the next morning.

This is the plunge that often that triggers that killer headache.

I've tried this and I can't say I noticed instant relief. But then again, I've suffered hangovers where my entire body feels like it's trying to run away from my brain, where the fires of hell could swallow me up and I'd still feel my head pounding. But as part of a general 'water and lying down' therapy, honey has certainly done the trick.

Better, and more instantly effective, is to drink a banana milkshake with honey. The banana and milk helps calm the stomach and rehydrate you, while the honey builds up the blood sugar levels. Bananas also contain electrolytes, magnesium and potassium, which are depleted during heavy drinking.

There's no specific recipe for this. Besides you'll be too hungover to read this book and measure out the amounts. So here's the gist:

> Chuck a load of bananas, ice and milk into a processor and give it a whizz. Add in honey to taste, then whizz again.

Job done. Now go and lie down.

Heartburn

Honey mixed with slippery elm is an effective remedy when your stomach is complaining about the amount you've stuffed in there.

Slippery elm is the powdered bark of a tree, native to North America. But it's available in many forms if you go to online health supplement websites (type 'slippery elm buy' into a UK-based search engine.)

The best way to take it is in tea form. You can buy it in powdered format, but watch out for ones with added sugar.

> Slippery elm has a thick consistency, so mix a teaspoon of it with a dash of cold water until it forms a smooth paste. Only then should you add boiling water and one or two teaspoons of honey.

You'll find even more on heartburn in PART THREE.

Hiccups

Okay, here's the deal. I've got a brilliant cure for hiccups that will amaze your friends and family. You absolutely must try it on one of your friends next time they have hiccups.

It's got absolutely *nothing* to do with honey. But if I got run over by a bus tomorrow and this cure died with me, I'd feel like I let humanity down. So I'll give you a popular honey-based tip first, then let you in on my secret.

> For hiccup problems, mix one teaspoon of vinegar (any type should do) and a couple of teaspoons of honey in a glass of warm water. Drink immediately. The sugar in the honey helps breaks up the hiccups.

Give it a go. Or try this Ray Collins Master Remedy (TM) instead.

> Get your hiccupping friend to put their fingers in their ears. Now fill a pint glass with water and tell them to drink most of the pint, taking consistent, tiny little sips. Talk them through it so they don't stop, and don't let them laugh or give up too early or the game's over.

When they stop sipping and remove their fingers, they will find their hiccups have gone.

This works 85% of the time for me. Each time, people gasp, "That's amazing. What are you, a *witch doctor?*"

"No," I say, "I'm just a writer".

And with that, I tip my hat, spin on my heels, and walk into the sunset.

Hirsutism (too much hair!)

It's one of the cruel ironies of life.

Men spend their young years desperate for manly hair to appear. It means we can finally shave like our dads, grow moustaches and fancy sideburns for the ladies. Then suddenly, before we know what's happening, we're old and desperate for the hair to stay on our heads. But it literally falls off us as we do the gardening and worry about interest rates.

Conclusion? Men love hair. But hair *hates* men.

And women? Well, you spend your lives thinking about your hair and colouring it, always wanting what you can't have. The curly girls want straight hair (remember the fashion for ironing hair in the '60s?) while the straight girls want wavy hair. Then, before you know it, you're in your later years and worrying about even *more* hair growing in unsightly, embarrassing places.

Conclusion? Women also love hair. But, even worse, hair loves women too.

Luckily, ladies, I've found a natural solution to the problem. You can try this honey and lemon-based mask to fade out that excess hair. The lemon will bleach while the honey soothes.

Mix a teaspoon of lemon juice with a teaspoon of honey. Smooth onto your face in the direction your hair is growing, and leave for ten minutes. Now you can rinse.

Excessive hair growth in women is known as 'hirsutism'. The problem is caused by male hormones, including testosterone. All women produce these chemicals, but when production gets excessive, unwanted extra hair can grow on your stomach, breasts and face.

In 2007, Turkish researchers discovered that extracts of spearmint plant were reducing the libido of men in Isparta, a town in southwest Turkey. They wondered whether it was reducing their male hormone levels. So they put it to the test on 21 women volunteers with hirsutism. They found a decrease in active testosterone in the blood and an increase in several female hormones.

They say it's early days yet, but it could be that drinking the tea twice a day can reduce the levels of male sex hormones in your body. Here's how to make a simple spearmint tea:

Pour 250ml of boiling water onto a heaped teaspoon of dried spearmint leaves. Add honey if you'd like a sweeter taste, (as well as the many other benefits of honey you'll see in this book). Leave it for 5-10 minutes, strain, and drink.

If you can't find spearmint leaves, look for pre-made spearmint tea at your local health food store, online, or even at your supermarket. A good quality tea with real spearmint leaves should be fine.

Indigestion/Ulcers

In the good old days, the "old wives" claimed that honey stirred into milk was a remedy for acid indigestion.

Why? The old wives didn't know, gawd bless 'em. It just worked.

And so millions of people dealt with their indigestion in a tasty, natural way. They were blissfully unaware of whether boffins in white coats thought it was "scientific" or not.

"It's an old wives' tale," the scientists declared, "and it shall remain so UNTIL WE SAY OTHERWISE!"

Then, hey presto, it happened.

Scientists have discovered that a bacteria called 'Helicobacter' is linked to acid indigestion and stomach ulcers, and that honey actually inhibits this bacteria.

Wow. Blow me down with a feather. The old wives were onto something after all.

But what the old wives may not have known is that *one* particular honey could do more than treat ulcers and indigestions. It could tackle the *causes* of these serious health problems.

Professor Peter Molan of the University of Waikato has found that strains of manuka honey can completely eradicate Helicobacter Pylori. And a preliminary clinical trial showed that ulcer patients who took 20 grams of manuka honey four times daily, one hour before meals and at bedtime, experienced less pain and discomfort than patients who took a honey with NO antibacterial activity.

If you haven't heard of manuka honey before, you should check it out. It's another odd tale of science struggling to catch up with nature.

Manuka honey comes from New Zealand. The local beekeepers set up their hives in wild areas in where manuka bushes grow. These bushes are indigenous only to New Zealand. On his adventures, Captain Cook used their leaves to make a tea with which he treated sailors with scurvy. This is why it's often called the 'tea tree'. The native Maoris also used it for a variety of ills and ailments.

According to Professor Molan, who has been pioneering the tests on this substance:

"In all honeys, there is – to different levels – hydrogen peroxide produced from an enzyme that bees add to the nectar. In manuka honey, and its close relative which grows in Australia called jelly-bush, there's something else besides the hydrogen peroxide."

He calls this the 'unique manuka factor', or 'UMF'.

We're catching on here in the UK. Manuka honey has been used on special dressings at the Manchester Royal Infirmary since May 2006. Dr Nick Slevin, a specialist at the hospital told the BBC:

"Manuka honey has special anti-inflammatory and anti-infection properties and is believed to reduce the likelihood of MRSA infection."

Not only is it resistant to bacterial strains like MRSA, but clinical trials at the Waikato Hospital have shown that UMF manuka honey has healing properties. It can be used to treat leg ulcers and pressure sores, which often occur when elderly patients with poor vascular systems are bedridden. This means it can help you heal after surgery.

To get hold of manuka honey, take a look on the internet. It's also found in most large supermarkets. If you go online you can also pick up sterilised manuka honey products like dressings and cream.

Yes, it's more expensive than regular honey. But don't think of it as a food, think of it as a medicine too.

For a quick indigestion remedy, make a cup of manuka honey and lemon tea, (two teaspoons of honey and the juice of a small lemon) adding some raw ginger slices and allowing it to sit for 10 minutes.

Inflammation

Have you ever read a book in which the author suggests that being stung is good for you? No, of course not. That would be ludicrous. Sheer madness. Weirder than a dog on a rocket.

Wouldn't it?

Well, not necessarily. This is one of those books. It's not my personal theory, but that of a small group of alternative practitioners and writers like Mihály Simics, author of **Bee Venom Therapy And Multiple Sclerosis** and Charles Mraz, author of **Health And The Honeybee.**

These people claim that there's a benefit to being stung. It's not the sting itself that's useful. It's the venom, which contains a large number of enzymes, peptides, amines, sugars, lipids and amino acids. The 'wow factor' ingredient is a substance called melittin, which just happens to be a powerful anti-inflammatory. This could have implications for sufferers of arthritis, tendon injuries, multiple sclerosis and hypertension.

Don't worry, I'm not suggesting you throw yourself onto a hive of bees, screaming "HEAL ME". You can benefit from the healing properties of bee venom, without the agony, by taking an oral mixture of bee venom and manuka honey. (For details on manuka honey, see the section on 'Indigestion'.)

These oral supplements are available online if you type 'bee venom product' into a search engine like www.google.com.

But please understand three things. Firstly there have been few scientific studies of bee venom, and results are inconclusive. Secondly, check you don't have an allergy to bee stings. And thirdly, make sure you consult your doctor before you try anything like this. For example, this type of product should NOT be taken if you suffer from cardiovascular disease, or if you're pregnant.

Memory

According to Dr Paul Gold of the University of Virginia, the energy boost from eating honey can improve your mind's ability to hold onto information. Much in the same way as a dose of caffeine in the morning is shown to boost concentration for a short period.

My tip?

> When you need to knuckle down and study, at home or work, make yourself a honey and lemon drink. Take the juice of a lemon, two teaspoons of honey and add some hot water.

Nappy rash

In studies reported in *Clinical Microbiology and Infection* in 2005, babies with nappy rash were treated with a topical mixture of honey, olive oil and beeswax.

This worked a treat, apparently. Although the babies didn't tell them this, they simply gurgled. It's a thankless task being a baby-based research scientist.

> Add a couple of teaspoons of honey to cooled-down camomile tea and use it to clean your baby's bottom. This should help clear up the nappy rash quickly.

Oily skin

This one isn't for the faint-hearted. And before you picture me covered in egg and honey, no I haven't tried it. This is one of those cases where I do the research, and you try it out.

Even if I did have oily skin, I don't know what I'd do if a mate came to the door and I answered it with this bizarre face pack on. Leave the country, perhaps. Or I'd go for a shock tactic and yell, "Thank god you've arrived!"

However, if you're up for it, here's what to do:

> Take a tablespoon of lemon juice and whisk it up with a teaspoon of set honey and two egg whites. Without laughing, spread the mixture on your face and leave for 20 minutes. Then rinse with water.

Honestly, I'm not making this up. *Would I do that to you?*

Scaly elbows

For dry, scaly elbows:

> Mix a teaspoon of vegetable oil with a teaspoon of lemon juice. Add a teaspoon of honey. Lovely. Now rub this into the offending elbows every day.

You should also try this after you've showered:

> Cut half a lemon and squeeze the juice out. Put a tiny bit of honey in the bottom of the lemon half. Now sit with your elbows in the lemon cups for 10 minutes. The acids in the lemon will exfoliate your skin, while they honey will help soothe and heal.

Sore throat

Does it feel like someone has sandpapered your throat? Here's what to do:

> Make a tea from fresh sage leaf, (purple or red sage works best) by adding half a litre of boiling water to a handful of sage leaves. When it's cooled slightly, add honey to taste. This will soothe and open up your throat. You can re-warm this mix and use it throughout the day.

One of my **Good Life Letter** readers says: "I recommended this to the singer Lisa Gerard (who contributed her voice to the Spartacus soundtrack) when she was having problems with her throat while touring."

Spots

You can heal your spots more quickly if you try this simply healing mask.

Add two teaspoons of honey to a quarter teaspoon of sea salt, plus a teaspoon of the spice turmeric. Mix into a thick paste. Apply to the spot before you go to bed and leave it overnight.

The next morning wash your face and hey presto, you should see a stark improvement.

Thirst

Ancient Egyptians supposedly took water with them on long journeys through the desert to stay hydrated. Honey packs an instant mineral punch to replenish your body's supplies.

To quench your thirst, mix two teaspoonfuls of honey in a large tumbler of water and knock it back. You should feel instant relief.

I realise you're not likely to be heading out into the desert as you read this. But I like to imagine that if you were, you'd take this book with you. Perhaps instead of a water canister.

Urination problems

The Koran recommended honey as a useful diuretic and laxative, which may even help you slim. I'll go into this in more detail in PART FOUR. Here's quick a method to try:

Pour 6 fluid ounces of freshly boiled water over 1 heaped tea-spoon of wild thyme (ideally the fresh stuff is best, but this also works with dried thyme). Cover and steep this mixture for three or four minutes. Strain and sweeten with honey.

Drink one cup of this tea daily.

Wrinkles

Do I have a problem with wrinkles? Certainly not. I've got plenty of them, thanks, and they keep coming every year. My wife thinks they make me look 'distinguished'.

That said, I also believe that Galapagos tortoises look quite distinguished.

Perhaps I should try a dose of my own anti-wrinkle medicine? Here are three versions of a classic natural remedy I've found:

1. Take 30 ml. of cabbage juice and mix it with a teaspoon of honey. Dab the mixture on your face every evening. To get the cabbage juice you'll need a juicing machine – oh, and a cabbage.

2. Mix a teaspoon of honey with a teaspoon of the cream you get from milk. Apply to your face, then wash after 20 minutes.

3. Take half a teaspoon of carrot juice. Then add one and half tablespoons of honey. Mix them up and apply to your face for twenty minutes before washing it off.

To see decent results, you should keep up any anti-wrinkle treatment every day for a period of 30 to 40 days at least.

CHAPTER THREE

The best honey to buy, and how to store it

As with most natural foods, the best kind of honey you can buy is the locally produced stuff. There are 35,000 beekeepers throughout the UK offering a wide range of honeys. So look for any beekeeping clubs in your area. The Internet is the best place to start your search. Or go to your local health food store and ask them for some advice.

When choosing your honey, you'll be faced with a range of options:

Whole comb – This is the unprocessed form of honey you get straight from the hive. You get big chunks of waxy comb immersed in raw honey. It doesn't store very well, so it won't last long in your cupboard. You will need to go to your local beekeeper to get this.

Raw – This is pretty much honey as it is, removed from the comb.

It's not heated or treated, and may contain bits of wax. Again, while it's very high in nutrients, this doesn't store very well. You can find this in health stores, farmers' markets, and some supermarkets. Or search online and you could get it delivered.

Filtered – To get rid of the particles and impurities you get in raw honey, the producer heats the honey. This is still good, natural stuff, though and stores well. Best of all, most of the vital nutrients are still in there. This is widely available anywhere.

Pure honey – This is the best honey for storing at home because it doesn't crystallise easily. It has been heated to higher temperatures to kill micro-organisms. This also means that it loses a lot of the vitamins that you need to benefit from the tips in this book.

Spun or crystallised – A lot of the moisture is removed to turn it into a creamy spread. This is the most processed type of honey, and the least beneficial in health terms.

To try out the many specialist international honeys, go online and use a search engine to find companies who can deliver to the UK. One of the best is manuka honey, from New Zealand, as I explain in the 'indigestion' section of this part of the book.

Manuka honey is now widely available in most supermarkets. But beware that not all are created equal. Some are more purified than others and exposed to higher levels of heat. For versions that maintain manuka honey's highly active properties, shop around online. Look for labels that say '10+ active' or above.

For beeswax and bee pollen products, you should definitely search online. There are countless bee product websites and shops in the UK now, supplying a whole range of products. Shop around for good deals, but remember that quality is key.

What colour honey is best?

As a guide, the lighter the colour of your honey, and the more delicate the flavour, the greater the price will be. My advice is to choose a good filtered honey that suits your taste, or go for the raw.

The ideal place to store the honey is a kitchen cupboard shelf or pantry shelf. Not the fridge.

Don't store honey near heat sources, or leave it in very cold places, as it will crystallise. If it does this, then heat a pan of water. While it's simmering, place the jar of honey in the pan for a few minutes, take it out and leave for another few minutes. Gently heated this way, the honey should melt slightly and become runnier.

Finally, when baking with honey, remember to reduce any liquid by a quarter of a cup for each cup of honey you use. Always add half a teaspoon of baking soda for each cup of honey you use. And reduce your oven temperature by 25°F to prevent the food from over-browning.

PART TWO

THE VAMPIRE'S NIGHTMARE
The antibacterial
wonder of garlic

CHAPTER ONE

A terrifying history of garlic

When I was a young boy, there were two things that terrified me. The first was the great white shark. This was thanks to the film *Jaws*, which came out in 1976 and lurked through my pre-adolescent mind like a reminder of death, until I discovered girls and music.

The second was the Triffid, the giant killer plant invented by the sci-fi writer John Wyndham. After reading *The Day of The Triffids* aged 9, I was convinced they were real. They were out there somewhere. Perhaps in the steaming depths of the Amazon jungle. And if so, they would surely come for us all one day.

I used to weigh up the pros and cons of being in certain places, depending on the shark-Triffid danger ratio. For instance, going to the beach was *bad*, because of the shark threat, and *good* because Triffids couldn't swim. Being inside the house was good, because of the lack of sharks; bad, because of the potential Triffid threat.

What I wasn't scared of was vampires. I'd seen the films with Christopher Lee and even dressed up as one at Halloween. Yes, I knew they could turn into bats. Yes, they could suck your blood. Yes, they could turn you into one of the undead.

But here's the thing: they were scared of garlic. What on earth was that all about?

To my young mind, this was ridiculous. It was like being able to fend off Jaws using a sprout. Or defeat an onslaught of Triffids with a bunch of dandelions. It took away all my fear. It meant that as long as I ate Italian food (the only food in those days where you found garlic, come to think of it) I was safe.

What I didn't realise at the time was the same reason for vampires fearing garlic would be the same reason I'd be writing passionately about it now, many years on.

Natural protection against disease

Among other things, the fictional vampire was a symbol of disease. The blood sucking trans-European beast stood for all those 19th century nasties, like syphilis, cholera and typhoid fever. Lots of these diseases were sexually transmitted (thus the seductive power of Dracula) or borne by mosquitoes (referenced by Dracula's blood-sucking antics).

For many centuries – long before Bram Stoker invented Dracula – garlic was considered one of the most powerful natural anti-bacterial and anti-fungal agents in the world. It can prevent disease, repel mosquitoes and keep your mind and body energised. It contains antioxidants which protect your body against the damaging free radicals which attack your cells and lead to cancer.

Best of all, the body doesn't seem to build up resistance to garlic so you can use it all your life to great effect.

In ancient Egyptian times they loved garlic so much they worshipped it. Clay models of garlic bulbs were discovered in the tomb of Tutankhamun. An Egyptian papyrus from 1,500 B.C. recommends garlic for 22 ailments. And some historians believe that the Egyptians fed it to slaves to increase their stamina as they built pyramids.

They even used garlic as a currency. At around 2,500 BC you could buy a decent slave for just 15 pounds of garlic. A bargain!

Prevent yourself turning into a pig

The ancient Greek poet, Homer wrote about how Ulysses avoided being changed into a pig with the help of garlic. This last one is a remedy I won't mention in this book. (If I ever come across a scientific study that shows how "pig-transformation" can be avoided with garlic, I'll let you know.)

More realistically, the classical Roman poet Virgil described how Thestylis used wild thyme and garlic as protection against snakebites. Certainly, it can clean wounds, as you'll discover in Chapter Two.

Hippocrates, the father of modern medicine, was a big fan of garlic, even more so than he was of honey (if you've read PART ONE, you know what I mean). He prescribed it for pretty much everything you can think of.

You could say he was hedging his bets.

In the Middle Ages it was commonly thought that garlic could prevent and even cure the plague. They prescribed garlic soup as medicine for victims of The Black Death. While I'm sure the garlic did some good, you can imagine the dying victim saying, "Okay, doctor, this looks absolutely lovely, really tasty. Now where's my cure?"

"That's your cure."

"This soup?"

"Yes, the soup."

"I think there's been a bit of confusion, Doc. I think I may need something a bit stronger... because, as you can see, I have THE PLAGUE!"

That said, it's not at all far-fetched that garlic could help you ward off serious disease. As part of your diet, many experts claim it can even help protect you from some cancers. In this part of the book, you'll discover that garlic is more powerful than most people realise.

Why garlic packs a punch

Packed into each pale clove is a heady cocktail of protein, vitamins A, B and C, and essential minerals including iron, calcium and selenium. All of these are vital for your good health. But the main reason for garlic's many super-powers is a chemical called allicin. This is the compound that also gives garlic its pungent smell.

Don't be put off by the whiff. This really is one of nature's wonders. When you crush a clove of garlic, allicin is quickly oxidized, releasing more than 100 biologically active compounds that can fight a whole host of viruses and infections.

Read on and you'll see what I mean...

CHAPTER TWO

The health benefits of garlic

Here are my favourite garlic remedies listed in alphabetical order. If you're interested in a specific ailment, and it's not here, remember the index at the back.

Acne

Acne is caused by an inflammation of the sebaceous glands and hair follicles on your face, neck, shoulders, back and chest. When these glands produce too much oil, the pores get clogged and show up as spots. Garlic is one of those home remedies that seems to work on this problem.

> For acne on your body, rub a clove of garlic over the problem area, and the blemish should disappear after a few days. But be very careful. Rub only a little, and lightly.

If you do this on your face it may burn, so instead take a crushed garlic clove, and mix it in a cup of warm water. Then you can gently apply the mixture to your face with a piece of clean cotton wool, avoiding the eyes.

I've read plenty of testimony to this from acne sufferers on many online forums. Some of them get over-excited and claim that it *cures* acne. It doesn't. But it can certainly help you control and ease the problem.

Asthma

The other day someone asked me if I enjoy 'surfing' the web. Certainly, as an alternative health writer, I use the Internet almost every day, foraging through forums and websites to see how every-day people treat common ailments like asthma.

A lot of forgotten knowledge is being swapped online, from country to country, culture to culture. The internet is a fantastic way to find those old remedies, recipes and ideas that have been handed down through generations.

But is 'surfing' the right word?

Surfing is term that means skimming the surface of something. It's a word for young people with few health worries, for those who want to zip through the social calendar, keep up with the times, and look better on the outside.

For them, the Internet is about using *Facebook* and *Myspace* to keep in touch. (Don't worry if you haven't got a clue what these things are, they're strange cyber-worlds populated by wannabe pop stars, bored office workers, and the under 30s!)

'How r u?' they ask each other.

'Gr8 thanx M8' they reply.

Then they promptly forward a short film of a cat playing the piano, a lion giving birth to a squirrel or a monkey dancing to ABBA.

While I'm going to admit right now that a giraffe stealing a bra is quite funny, I think of myself less as a 'surfer' and more as a scubadiver. I probe deep for pearls of health information that you won't find in flash-technology websites, online newspapers, or bandied about on trendy social networks. Stuff which you will find *useful*. Recommendations, tips and recipes that real people swear by. Simple, workable ways to make yourself feel fitter and happier inside.

And not a lip-synching monkey in sight.

In the case of asthma, there's so much to learn from people's experiences. From scouring websites and forums, based across the planet, from Bolivia to India, I've found testimony to garlic's effectiveness in helping sufferers deal with asthma the natural way.

There's no one 'cure-all' recipe. But here are three versions I've culled from my Internet scubadiving:

1. Boil three cloves of peeled and crushed garlic in 120 millilitres of vinegar. After cooling this mixture, strain it and add an equal quantity of honey. Mix and put in a sealed jar. Take one or two teaspoons of this syrup in the evening and before going to bed.

2. Chop 3 cloves of garlic into smaller chunks. Let them steep in a large glass of milk overnight. Make sure the fridge is very cool to avoid any unwanted organisms growing off your garlic. The next day, drink it down, or take a tablespoon of the mix every three hours.

For a quicker version of the above, you can boil the chopped garlic in the milk, let it cool slightly and then drink it before you go to bed.

3. Slice some raw ginger (six or seven slices off the root will do it) into hot water, along with a two cloves of minced garlic, and leave this to steep for 10 minutes. Drink this in the morning and then again before you for to bed

If you suffer from asthma, please be sure to talk to a medical professional. Find out the root causes of your problem and make sure an allergy to specific types of foods isn't the problem. If you're allergic to milk for instance, recipe number 2 isn't going to help at all.

Athlete's Foot

In my early twenties I lived in a small flat in Cardiff with my brother. Our bathroom was tiny and without a ventilation fan. Its carpeted floor was permanently soggy. Tiny mushrooms grew between the cracks of the tiles.

Yes, it's disgusting, I know. But this was long before my transformation into a health obsessive. At that time I was a young man with an office job, a love of post-work beers, and no time for a rigorous morning regime.

Every day I'd wake up late, my hair like an electric hedge. In a panic, I'd stumble from my bed, into the shower, across the sodden carpet, into my clothes, out the door and onto the bus in approximately 5 minutes.

Unsurprisingly, I developed athlete's foot. The fungus spread between my toes, across my soles and heels. It was very hard to shift. I bought a chemical spray that burned my feet, filled my bedroom with an acrid mist, and didn't work.

One morning I was so tired, I mistook the can of fungal foot spray for my deodorant and blasted it into my armpits. Not recommended.

All this expense and misery would have been unnecessary if I'd known what I do today. The allicin in garlic is famously anti-fungal and antibiotic, making it an instant and inexpensive solution for athlete's foot.

There are a few ways to tackle the problem:

The first method is to rub a clove of raw garlic straight onto the affected area.

Or put some freshly crushed garlic on the affected area, cover it with a bandage and leave it for half an hour. Simply wash with water afterwards.

Do this once a day for a week and the athlete's foot should be gone. If you get a horrible burning sensation, then take it all off, wash it with water and try again. This time, use crushed garlic steeped in a little water.

If it's still not right for you, go for an even milder approach. Add some surgical spirit and 6 cloves of crushed garlic to a big basin of warm water. Now stick your feet in there and give them a soak. Put the telly on, read a book.

If anyone asks what you are doing, reply "I'm being athletic."

Blood pressure

In 1994, clinical trials published in the *Journal of the Royal College of Physicians* showed that taking garlic tablets reduced volunteers' blood pressure between 1% and 5%.

Why? Well, Ajoene, a compound found in garlic, is said to stop your blood from clotting. The authors of the report reckoned this could cut the incidence of stroke by 30% to 40%, and heart disease by 20% to 25%.

In 1997, published research from the University of Alabama went a step further. They showed that the allicin in garlic reacts with red blood cells to produce hydrogen sulphide. This also relaxes the blood vessels and eases the strain on your heart.

Ever heard of homocysteine? It's the stuff that can damage the blood vessel lining, which can lead to fatty deposits in your arteries. The vitamin B6 in garlic keeps these homocysteine levels low.

A study of adults aged 50 to 80 also found that garlic could prevent your body's main artery, the aorta, from stiffening with age. When this occurs, the aorta has trouble opening and closing.

"Working that hard causes the heart, like any muscle, to become bigger and thicker, which makes it more prone to failure," says John Streitman, M.D. a cardiac surgeon at FirstHealth Moore Regional Hospital.

Easing the strain on your heart is not the only line of defence that garlic offers. It contains selenium and manganese, powerful antioxidants that can protect the heart from damage after surgery.

These antioxidants may help to lower blood cholesterol levels, too. However, there's a lot of debate about this. A study published in the Archives of Internal Medicine in 2007 said that garlic did NOT lower bad levels of cholesterol. Even so, the researcher for that project, Christopher Gardner, conceded that it was possible that garlic could lower levels when taken at higher doses, or in people with higher cholesterol levels.

Even the sceptics are sceptical about their scepticism. So in my view, the jury is still out on this. Many experts remain convinced about the link between high garlic intake and low levels of bad cholesterol.

At this point, I'd love to offer you a 'one-stop' instant remedy for high blood pressure. You could follow the simple instructions, perhaps a quick recipe for soup, and become disease-free in five minutes.

If only the world worked that way!

The truth is, it's a matter of changing your lifestyle. Take a holistic approach. Cut out processed foods and lower your alcohol intake. Eat a balanced diet and do some exercise. And include plenty of raw garlic in your diet every day. Grate it into salads, or put it into the juicer with lots of carrot, orange and apple.

You should also try the daily garlic and ginger tea in the "asthma" section above. Or look for supplements at your health store.

One final thing on this subject. If you are worried about high blood pressure or your cholesterol levels, please get yourself checked out by a doctor. Oh, and be aware that garlic thins the blood. This may make it dangerous to take before serious operations.

Cancer

Don't panic, I'm not about to start trumpeting a garlic cure for cancer. Nothing of the sort. I'll leave that to the many snake-oil salesmen out there, who prey on people's desperation with magic potions and false hope.

Instead, I'd like to show you some of the incredible discoveries science has made regarding garlic's ability to prevent serious disease.

Yes, and this primarily involves the 'C' word.

The first modern scientific study of garlic's effect on cancer happened in the 1950s, when a bunch of scientists injected allicin into mice with cancer. The treated mice survived more than six months whereas those who didn't get the injection managed only two.

When it comes to prostate and stomach cancers, there's certainly some recent evidence that allicin and other ingredients in garlic can help you in the fight.

Research by a team from the University of North Carolina at Chapel Hill, found that people who eat raw or cooked garlic regularly cut their risk of stomach cancer by about a half. One reason is that the anti-bacterial properties of garlic make it effective against a bacterium called Helicobacter pylori. (See PART ONE – **'Indigestion and Ulcers'** for more details.) This is found in the stomach and is known to promote cancer. Another reason is that the allyl sulfur compounds in garlic could slow the growth of tumour cells.

In China, researchers have found that smokers who eat lots of garlic have a relatively lower stomach cancer risk than smokers who don't. Even more remarkably, men in China have the lowest rate of prostate cancer in the world.

Could this be related to their diet, which is very high in onions, garlic and shallots?

This is the claim in a study from the *Journal of the National Cancer Institute*. Researchers asked men from Shanghai how often they ate certain foods. Those men who ate more than a third of an ounce each day from the allium foods – namely garlic, shallots and onions – were 50% less likely to have prostate cancer.

And in the USA, a Women's Health Study in Iowa showed that middle-aged women who regularly consumed garlic had 35% lower risk of developing colon cancer.

These trials continue, of course. But certainly in terms of serious disease prevention, it would do no harm to begin adding garlic to your daily diet. Any of the recipes and methods in this book will work well.

Take a look at my specific recommendations in the section 'Blood pressure'.

Coughs and colds

I don't know who gets paid to sit in an office and come up with weird statistics, but they must be out there somewhere, tapping on an enormous calculator. The latest one I've heard is that average British person spends about two to three years of his life with a cold.

That's two hundred colds for the average 75-year-old man.

Who knows how much this costs the UK economy? Although it *does* boost viewing figures for daytime television, sales of tissues, and the profits of the big drug companies who supply cold and flu remedies.

As you've seen from the chapter on honey, there's really no need to waste your money on these expensive artificial remedies. As the BBC reported back in October 2001, garlic could help *prevent the common cold!*

You may groan with disbelief. But this was the claim from team of researchers led by Peter Josling, director of the Garlic Centre in East Sussex. They found that taking a garlic supplement each day makes people less likely to fall victim to a cold. It's that good old allicin, again, releasing compounds that act as a powerful antibacterial agent, fighting off infections that attack your body.

To explain this quickly, what happens when you get a cold is that an organism called a rhinovirus invades your body. Once it's got its claws (or its big horn, I suppose) into you, the virus replicates itself more than 100,000 times, spreading through your body. Next thing you know, you're either watching Jeremy Kyle from underneath a pile of tissues, or spattering mucus over your work colleagues.

It takes your body a lot of work to fight off this cold once you have it. Really all you can do is manage the situation. So the real secret is to avoid the rhinovirus charging into your system in the first place. Which is where garlic comes into its own.

Studies found that daily garlic supplements can reduce the risk of catching a cold by half. It's a powerful preventative. So the best way to use garlic to fight a cold is to take it as soon as your work colleagues or loved ones start coming down with it.

Even if you *do* catch the lurgie from that annoying bloke in accounts, it can help you fight the symptoms and relieve your stuffy nose.

For coughs and flu, you should make this simple homemade cough syrup:

> Slice a pound of fresh garlic and pour a litre of boiling water over it. Let it sit for 12 hours. Now add two tablespoons of cider vinegar, bring it to the boil and gradually add sugar until it becomes syrupy. Add honey to taste. Then cool. Now take a teaspoon of this mixture three times a day, or whenever necessary.

For your sore throat:

> Steep seven cloves of garlic in half a cup of water overnight. The next morning, drink it down in a few gulps.

It's not exactly as luxurious as your morning coffee, but it should offer you some relief.

Earache

If you're suffering from earache, use a blender to crush a clove of garlic into three tablespoons of olive oil until it's completely smooth. Lie down on your bed and have your loving partner put three drops down your ear.

Really, my wife LOVES doing this. There's nothing that rekindles a romance more than pouring fluids into ears.

Anyway, put on the radio, like back and stay like this for half an hour. Make it as easy as possible on yourself. Repeat this little ritual twice a day. Hey, you may even start pretending you have earache so you get to lie down and have some peace from time to time.

I won't tell if you won't.

Impotency

In ancient China and Japan, the people believed that garlic could boost energy, lift bad moods, and improve male potency.

So was this superstition?

After all, history is littered with the corpses of debunked aphrodisiacs. Take the classic Arab book, *The Perfumed Garden*, for example. This old sexual advice manual recommended a pill that contained, among other things, magpie poo. In Elizabethan times they thought the humble potato as an aphrodisiac and called them "Apples of Love".

In the 21st century, little has changed. If I see another piece of spam mail offering me the elixir of sexual performance from a "combination of secret ingredients", I'll scream. Especially when a more effective remedy is there in your local supermarket or corner shop for a matter of pennies.

With garlic, there's good evidence for its powers in the bedroom. For many men, the problem of erectile dysfunction comes down to inefficient blood flow caused by a hardening of the arteries. As you've already seen in the section on 'blood pressure', garlic can improve the flow of blood.

So in these cases, garlic could work.

In 2007 a BBC TV programme called The Truth About Food took seven volunteers with erectile dysfunction and told them to eat four garlic cloves a day. Six out of seven of the group saw a marked improvement in the bedroom.

A small test, perhaps, but it won't do you any harm to try it. The only side effect is bad breath, something I'll deal with in Chapter Three.

Of course, if the problem is psychological one, then no substance will help. In this case, please talk to a professional who can counsel you, or give you sound advice. And throw that junk mail 'Make love like a 21 year old GUARANTEED' thing away. It's bunkem.

Unless you happen to be a 21-year-old.

Infections

The famous French microbiologist Louis Pasteur discovered the anti-bacterial power of garlic back in 1858.

Well, actually, this isn't strictly true. The Ancient Egyptians discovered it when they used garlic as medicine. As did the Ancient Greeks, the Chinese and the Indians.

Okay, so Pasteur first proved garlic's anti-bacterial power *in a laboratory*. He put some garlic cloves in a petri dish containing bacteria. A few days later he found that the garlic had killed the surrounding bacteria. The word was out! And just over 55 years later World War One surgeons were regularly using garlic poultices to stop wounds turning septic.

A heap of studies show that garlic can kill many bacteria, including Escherichia, Salmonella, Staphylococcus, Streptococcus, Klebsiella, Proteus, Bacillus, and Clostridium – all the ones that sound like dinosaurs or Roman gods. In total, garlic is credited with killing 23 types of bacteria.

It's a veritable *germ murderer.*

In modern times, many nasty strains of bacteria have become resistant to antibiotics. Now our hospitals are plagued by life-threatening superbugs. But lots of them, like E Coli, can be destroyed by the allicin in garlic.

In 2003, Dr Ron Cutler and his team at the University of East London discovered that allicin can cure MRSA "within weeks". It even destroys the newer strains that cannot be treated by Vancomycin and Glycopeptides, dubbed the 'last line of defence' antibiotics.

This is why Garlic can quickly and cleanly cure nasty boils on your leg or arm, as well as other minor wounds. Here's a version of the World War I method you can try at home.

> First, use a garlic press or juicer to get the juice from some fresh garlic cloves. Apply the juice to the boil or infected wound. Now cover with a loose bandage until the head of the boil begins to soften.

> Take off the compress when the head of the boil has softened. Remove the head and clean the wound with warm distilled or purified water. Pour more juice into the wound to disinfect it.

> Now wash it all out again with clean water and bandage yourself up. Remember to change the dressing twice a day.

Insect repellent

Apart from a predilection for biting women, vampires and mosquitoes have something else in common: they both hate garlic.

Garlic contains Diallyl disulfide and diallyl trisulfide, two compounds that can kill mosquito larvae and repel all kinds of insects, including fleas and black flies. It works if you spray garlic oil on your body, and also if you eat it. When you ingest garlic, the repellent compounds are released through your skin and mouth.

Yes, you too can have breath that wards off insects. *Roll up, roll up!*

There are two ways you can go about this. First is to make your own all-natural insect repellent spray.

> Get some garlic oil and mix with 5 parts water. Buy a cheap spray bottle from your local garden centre and fill with the smelly water. Shake well and spray on your body or around the most affected parts of the home to get protection for up to six hours.

Another method is to melt some beeswax, add an equal amount of petroleum jelly, and then add some garlic oil. You can then rub this onto your skin. This is much better than dousing yourself with DEET and other outrageous chemicals that you get in artificial repellents.

Low energy

Garlic has a long history as a performance-enhancing 'pick-me-up'. It was handed out like a legal drug to the Olympic athletes in Ancient Greece. Early Greek soldiers were also given garlic to eat before going into battle. It's something you never think about when you imagine those violent clashes between the Greeks and Trojans. The smell of garlic breath must have been atrocious. Mind you, it's a good incentive to chop people's heads off.

To give yourself a modern energy boost with this juice, have a go at one of my tried and tested recipes:

> Take four carrots, a chunk of ginger, two oranges, and a clove of garlic. Put them into a juicer and whizz it up. Pour over crushed ice and drink.

Now sprint off into the distance to do whatever it is you need to do.

Poisoning

Garlic can increase the activity of several enzymes in your liver, such as glutathione-S-transferase and cytochrome P450. These help your body clean out poisons and toxins.

For example, scientists have found that garlic may be helpful in cases of chronic lead poisoning. After being fed garlic cloves, animals that had been exposed to high levels of lead had significantly less of it in their livers than animals who didn't eat the garlic.

Garlic can increase the rate at which your body rids itself of other toxic metals, like cadmium and mercury.

In January 2008, *The New Scientist* revealed that garlic helps millions of Bangladeshis and Indians stave off combat arsenic contamination in their drinking water. Keya Chaudhuri of the Indian Institute of Chemical Biology in Kolkata, found that rats that were fed garlic extracts had 40% less arsenic in their blood and liver, and passed 45% more arsenic in their urine.

She advises taking one to three cloves of garlic per day as a preventative measure.

Sinus headaches

If your headache is one of those where you get a dull face ache around the eyes, cheeks, and jaw, and it feels worse when you move your head, there's a good chance that this is sinus related. To shift it, make a tea from garlic and ginger.

Take two cloves of garlic and two slices of fresh ginger. Steep them in hot water for ten minutes then and drink, breathing the steam through your nose.

Skin infections

As you now know, garlic has amazing anti-fungal powers. Not only can it treat athlete's foot, but it can also help with other fungal skin infections.

Smear some honey on the affected area and leave it for 15 minutes. Wash it off and pat the area dry. Next, apply some crush garlic cloves and do the same thing.

Try this twice a day.

Stomach bugs

If someone in your house picks up a stomach bug, eat two large garlic cloves. The virus will run into a brick wall. Garlic will kill any intestinal bacteria and help you produce more acid-producing bacteria to fight infection.

Be warned. If you take garlic by chewing it up, it tends to burn the mouth. Instead, finely chop up the clove (one 2 times a day is way plenty) and let it sit for 10 minutes before putting it in a teaspoon. Then wash it down with a glass of water.

It is now almost tasteless and won't repeat on you too much.

Stuffy nose

Crush the small end of a garlic clove and use it like a Vick's inhaler. Breathe the fumes in through your nostrils. This will help clear the passages and fight the germs.

Toothache

This one may surprise you. Garlic is a fantastic remedy for toothache. I realise I've mentioned Hippocrates a lot in this book, but you can't knock the master. Back in 400 BC he was happily recommending garlic to patients with toothache. Although, as I've already said, he hedged his bets by prescribing garlic for everything he was faced with. It was his default setting.

You can imagine life in the Hippocrates surgery...

"Doctor, my hand has been cut off in a fight."

"Have you tried garlic?"

But he was onto something with his toothache theory. It works. The quickest method is to gently crush a clove of garlic, but so that it still remains in one lump, and put it on between the tooth and gum.

If you're having gum problems, garlic is a clever option to try. In a 2005 study published in *Archives of Oral Biology*, researchers claimed that garlic extract can kill disease-causing bacteria in your mouth. This can help you fight off gum diseases like periodontitis.

CHAPTER THREE

How to grow, use and store garlic

People who grow their own garlic swear that it's far tastier than anything you can buy. It's quite easy to cultivate some in your own garden. You should buy your bulbs from proper seed merchants or garden centres. This will make sure that they are virus-free and specially bred for growing locally.

Plant the cloves in midwinter so you can harvest them the following summer. Choose an area of your garden that gets lots of sun and where the soil is not too damp. Prepare the soil two months before you plant the garlic, by digging it over and adding manure. Now plant the garlic about 2 and a half centimetres beneath the surface, and ten centimetres apart.

You'll find that the garlic takes about 6 months to grow. For every clove you plant you'll get a tasty bulb. As it reaches maturity, the leaves die away which is your signal to dig them up and dry them out.

If, like most people, you decide not to bother with all that, buy garlic from the shops instead.

Pick fat cloves and avoid the elephants

At the grocer, always pick garlic bulbs with firm, fat cloves. Look for dry skin and avoid those with shoots.

You may come across very large garlic bulbs, called 'elephant garlic'. This is actually closer to the leek than garlic and has a much milder flavour. Critics say that it's garlic "for people who don't like garlic". I would stick to the real thing to get the full benefits of the tips and remedies in this book.

Yes, you can buy garlic in bottles and tubes. This is fine for your convenience when cooking, but to get the most out of this book, get the fresh stuff.

As soon as you've got them home, store your garlic bulbs in a cool, dry, dark place. Unbroken garlic bulbs will keep for three to four months, while the individual cloves will hang around from for about a week only. Best to keep it all together, then.

Don't panic if you see green shoots poking out of your garlic after a few weeks. It doesn't mean that it's beyond redemption, or that you'll eat it and a tree will grow out of your head. It will have a milder flavour, that's all.

There's not much point in freezing your garlic. If you want it to keep for ages, then pickle it in wine or vinegar. Stick this in the fridge and your pickled garlic will be okay for three months.

Unless you know what you're doing, it's best not to store your garlic in oil as there have been reported cases of botulism in the past. This is because the sulphur in garlic makes it a potential breeding ground. Never store raw garlic in oil at room temperature, and never let it outstay its welcome in the fridge.

A warning

While I'm on the subject, some people have allergic reactions to garlic, or low tolerance. This can result in a bit of heartburn or flatulence. So if you notice any side effects from eating garlic, go and talk to your doctor or get an allergy test.

Health officials say that you shouldn't eat garlic for up to ten days before you're scheduled for surgery. This is because garlic thins the blood, which could cause problems. Again, if you are worried about any of this, please talk to a medical professional.

Remember that allicin is very strong, so don't eat more than 3 cloves of raw garlic a day. Otherwise you could irritate your stomach. This is a strong natural medicine, so don't go overboard.

Follow this '15-minute rule'

You'll still get some of the health benefits if you cook with garlic. But for the best medicinal effect, peel the garlic and let it sit for fifteen minutes before you cook with it, or make your teas and concoctions. Then crush it and use it immediately.

Lots of trendy chefs like Jamie Oliver just chuck in garlic with the papery skin still on, but for the maximum health benefits, take it off.

Unlike my good self, it's better in the nude.

Don't peel or crush the garlic days in advance of using it. The all-powerful allicin will react with the air and by the time you eat it, the beneficial properties will have faded. Oh, and when you're cooking with onion and garlic, chuck in the onion first. It takes longer to cook. Toss the garlic in later to avoid it burning and tasting bitter.

And finally, let me address this big question...

"How do I stop myself stinking of garlic?"

Come on, admit it, you've been reading this part of the book and wondering, right?

Well, I'll admit that garlic therapy can be a little, let's say, *aromatic*. And there's not much you can do. One way of lessening the problem is to chomp on some fresh parsley after you've eaten garlic. After you've hit the parsley, brush your teeth and all should be well.

You can also use garlic supplements. These work well. Make sure you check the label for the amount of allicin, as this is the really important chemical. The most portent versions have up to 5,000 micrograms (mcg) of allicin.

Not all supplements are of the same standard, so don't automatically go for the cheaper option.

PART THREE

HANNIBAL'S SECRET WEAPON
The surprising power of vinegar

CHAPTER ONE

A surprising history of vinegar

Before I launch into this chapter, I'll admit it. I'm about to exhibit the 'boring Dad' behaviour that can drive my children screaming from the dinner table. But in the same way as stretch elastic trousers really *are* more comfortable when you're lazing about the house, there is a point to my little history question.

And that question is: What was the most surprising thing about General Hannibal's famous surprise attack on the Romans in 218 BC?

Many people who studied this at school will immediately answer: "He travelled across the mountains *on elephants*."

And yes, it's true. The Carthaginian General *did* catch the Romans off-guard by crossing the Pyrenees and the Alps with 50,000 infantry troops, 9000 cavalry troops and 37 elephants. I imagine anyone in Northern Italy in 218 BC would have been extremely surprised by the sight of an African pachyderm trundling down the mountain. Even if their first reaction was, "That fat horse has a massive nose."

Or whatever that translates to in Latin.

To me, this wasn't the most surprising element of the story. What is far more surprising is that Hannibal used *vinegar* to crack open the rocks so that his troops, horses and elephants could get through tricky mountain passes.

We know this amazing fact thanks to the writings of the Roman historian Titus Livius. He described how Hannibal's soldiers chopped down trees, stacked them against the rock and set fire to the pile of wood, channelling the wind to fan the flames.

In **The History of Rome Vol. III** he says: "When the rock was red hot they poured vinegar upon it to disintegrate it. After thus treating it by fire they opened a way through it with their tools, and eased the steep slope by winding tracks of moderate gradient, so that not only the baggage animals but even the elephants could be led down."

You've got to hand it to Hannibal. This was one of the most dramatic uses of vinegar in history. But vinegar has had an illustrious role in the story of mankind.

A whirlwind tour of vinegar's healing past

Back in 5000 BC, the Babylonians used vinegar as a pickling agent. As with honey and garlic, there is evidence of widespread vinegar use in ancient Egypt. Our old friend Hippocrates, who has starred heavily in all three parts of this book, was also a fan of vinegar. In Ancient Greece he could be found prescribing it for skin rashes, coughs and colds.

Vinegar even appears in the bible. After working gleaning barley in the fields, Ruth is invited by Boaz to eat bread and dip it in vinegar. (Ruth 2:14) And according to the gospels of Matthew and Mark, Jesus was offered vinegar while on the cross.

While Hannibal was using vinegar to smash up rocks, his Roman enemies were drinking it in the form of 'posca'. This popular tipple was made from vinegar diluted with water and sweetened with honey. They drank it for an energy boost. And because the vinegar purified the dodgy drinking water.

During the U.S. Civil War, soldiers used vinegar to prevent stomach upsets and as a treatment for pneumonia and scurvy. And, as with honey, vinegar was another important battlefield medicine in World War I, acting as a readily available antiseptic.

From the urns of the Pharaohs, to the mountains of southern Europe to the Somme, vinegar has an eclectic history.

So what is vinegar?

The word comes from the Old French term *vin aigre*, meaning 'sour wine'. And that's pretty much what it is. In the late 19th century, the microbiologist Louis Pasteur found that if you add oxygen, yeast and bacteria to wine, the alcohol breaks down into acetic acid. This is vinegar. His famous pasteurisation process allowed this to become a commercial, industrialised product for export and widespread use.

As you'll see in Chapter Three, vinegar comes in many varieties. It can be made from almost any food that contains natural sugars. Yeast ferments the sugars into alcohol, and bacteria turn that alcohol into vinegar. For instance, you get white vinegar from distilled alcohol. Wine and cider vinegar come from grapes and apples. You can also oxidise malted barley or oats to get malt vinegar.

In Europe, we don't really sell vinegar on the basis that it's healthy. Here in Britain most people see it as something smelly and bad for you that goes on chips. If you're a fan of home cooking, no doubt you have a selection of vinegars to use as dressings and marinades.

But over in Japan, vinegar-based health drinks are huge business. The country's largest vinegar maker, Mizkan Group, says the market for vinegar drinks has grown from 7.57 billion yen between March and August 2000 to a whopping 21.46 billion yen between March and August 2004.

In 2005, *Guardian* journalist Justin McCurry visited Uchibori's Oaks Heart stall, which sells flavoured vinegars in Tokyo. In his report, he interviewed Satoko Higuchi, one of the sales staff who said:

"I get through a bottle a week. I usually mix it with mineral water and carry it around with me in a plastic bottle. It's great if you're on a diet and it seems to be doing my skin some good. My four-year-old daughter was practically raised on the stuff."

This is the kind of testimony you get from people who have converted to vinegar as an aid to healthy living. It's impressive how passionate these advocates are, and how much anecdotal evidence there is for vinegar's many benefits.

And no amount of sneering by sceptics will put them off.

While many ridicule vinegar fans for their 'lack of science', this hasn't stopped people since the Babylonian times using it to improve their lives.

As you're about to see, vinegar is not a wacky alternative medicine. It's not the latest fad. It's something that people have used for thousands of years, long before modern science. What follows is my investigation into the many ways people use vinegar to treat everyday ailments.

I'll leave you to be the judge.

CHAPTER TWO

The health benefits of vinegar

My friends may call me a "predictable old information junkie", but yet again I've gone listed all the ailments that vinegar could help *in alphabetical order*. I can't help it. I've got an addiction to putting things in order. My therpist says its okay.

Here I go again...

Allergies

According to the charity, *Allergy UK*, many household chemicals found in bleach and air fresheners can cause the symptoms of allergies.

"We don't have any official figures for the number of people, allergy sufferers or otherwise, affected by household chemicals," says Muriel Simmons, chief executive. "What we do know is that many asthma sufferers are sensitive to chemicals in cleaning products."

These chemicals include Benzene, which is found in paints, varnishes and solvents. It can cause irritation of eyes, nose, skin and throat, as well as dizziness, high heartbeat, vomiting and headaches. Trichloroethylene, which you get in household cleaners, can cause fatigue and dizziness. The ammonia in window cleaner can irritate your skin, eyes and lungs. Pesticides can affect your skin, eyes, nervous system and digestive tract.

And those lovely, cutesy air fresheners that you see advertised on TV by cartoon woodland animals? They contain volatile organic compounds (VOCs), which some studies suggest can cause asthma in children.

The implications are grim, and who knows what further research will reveal.

One of the ways to reduce these allergic reactions is to avoid using so many of these artificial cleaners and fresheners. Instead, turn to vinegar. It's a powerful all-natural household cleaner that has no irritants or side-effects.

Here are some ways you can use it to replace all those expensive sprays:

- To repel ants, spray vinegar around the doors, skirting boards and other places where the ants appear.

- To clean windows and mirrors, add a couple of tablespoons of vinegar to a small bucket of warm water, wash, then dry with a clean cloth. Or pour a quarter of a cup of vinegar into a spray bottle and top it up with water.

- You can also take the above mixture and spray it lightly into a room to freshen the air. Or fill a small bowl with vinegar and leave it in the room for a few hours. It will get rid of the smell of cigarette smoke. If something really has been stinking up the house, boil 3 tablespoons of vinegar in a cup of water. Alternatively, simmer cinnamon sticks or cloves in a pot of water.

- To shine brass and copper, dissolve a teaspoon of salt in a cup of distilled vinegar and rub that onto the stain.

- Clean your dishwasher by adding a cup of vinegar to the machine and running it through a complete cycle.

- To unclog drains, pour in a cup of baking soda then add half a cup of vinegar, then sluice out with hot water.

- Wash your fridge with a mixture of equal parts water and vinegar.

- Clean soap scum and mildew from showers, baths and sinks by wiping the surface with vinegar. Now rinse with warm water.

- To make your own cleaning mixture for the toilet, sprinkle a cup of borax around the toilet bowl. Ask about borax at your local chemist, or check out Boots, which have their own brand. Next, pour half a cup of white distilled vinegar around the bowl. Leave this for six hours, then scrub as you would normally.

- Clean your woodwork with this mix: one cup of ammonia, half a cup of vinegar, and a quarter of a cup of baking soda.

- For greasy pots and pans, soak the dirty items water along with two teaspoons of baking soda and a little vinegar.

- For clothes, add a quarter of a cup of vinegar to your washing machine's rinse cycle. This will make sure the detergent is rinsed from your clothes, helping avoid that scratchy, itchy feeling you sometimes get.

I'm not saying you need to go all-natural overnight, but some of these simple alternatives could provide a much healthier home for you and your family.

It's worth a shot, isn't it?

Asthma

If you suffer from asthma, you'd be well advised to follow the tips in the above 'allergies' section. By avoiding all the irritants in household cleaners and fresheners, you may find your problems easing a little.

There's also an old home remedy you can try if you get an attack. Try applying a hot apple cider vinegar compress over your entire chest area.

> To make the compress, take a piece of clean gauze, muslin, linen, or cotton and lay it out flat. Pour vinegar onto the cloth. Now place another cloth on top. Then place the compress over your chest. When the compress loses its heat, wash your body with water. Replace the cloths every 15 minutes, or whenever cool.

If you can't lie down to put it on your chest, apply the hot vinegar compress on your stomach and walk around the room for ten minutes.

Bad breath

There can be many reasons for bad breath. They include smoking, the taking of certain drugs and medications, dietary changes, gum disease, dehydration, zinc deficiency, stomach problems or serious illness.

If you get persistent bad breath and nothing solves it, you should get yourself checked out by a doctor. There could be a serious underlying condition.

Mostly, bad breath is caused by the bacteria that help you break down food in your mouth. Sometimes they begin to release smelly compounds. So if you've been unusually unpopular at parties, or people choose to sit farther away from you in meetings at work, you may want to check out the bad breath factor. Simply cup your hands over your mouth and nose, breathe out and then sniff.

If you feel like keeling over, or as if Beelzebub himself is breathing fire into your eyeballs, then you may want to try the following procedure.

> Dilute half a tablespoon of the vinegar into a glass of water and gargle it in your mouth for 10 seconds. Then rinse your mouth. You should also drink eight glasses of water through-out the rest of the day to wash away the germs and bacteria.

Beware that regular drinking of pure vinegar can harm the enamel on your teeth. So always drink it with water and rinse afterwards. Don't brush your teeth immediately after a vinegar treatment. Wait for at least half an hour.

For an instant remedy, chew fresh parsley leaves (as recommended in PART TWO for garlic breath) then brush your teeth.

Another reason for bad breath could be that you don't have enough stomach acid to digest your food properly. Many people believe that vinegar can behave like stomach acid and give your digestive powers a boost.

> To try this, take a tablespoon of vinegar in a glass of water half an hour before lunch. Or simply add vinegar to your meals in the form of a dressing (more about this in Chapter Three).

Be wary of gargling with undiluted apple cider vinegar, as it can burn your throat.

Bad hair and dandruff

Hair is mildly acidic. But many of the hair care products on sale are strongly alkaline. So rinsing with apple cider vinegar can help balance the pH of your hair and remove the build-up that can result from using alkaline products. It can also help you fight dandruff.

Give it a go and see if your hair becomes shinier, smoother and easier to manage. It may smell a tad 'vinegary' after rinsing, but once dry this should disappear completely.

> Make your own healthy after-shampoo hair rinse mixing a tablespoon of apple cider vinegar with 1 cup (250 ml) of warm filtered tap water.

Bee stings

This one is simple. If you get stung, immediately rub vinegar onto the affected area. Job done. If you haven't already, go back and read PART ONE for a bizarre health remedy involving bee stings.

Blood pressure

I've read many anecdotal reports online, and had plenty of emails from readers of my newsletter *The Good Life Letter*, suggesting that apple cider vinegar could help control blood pressure. In my view this is a folk remedy and not some blanket miracle 'cure' in all cases.

For instance, it can work for people who have too much protein in their diet. When you have too much protein, your blood can become more alkaline, which makes it thicker. This can lead to a rise in blood pressure. The acid in the vinegar could work to counter this by thinning your blood and making it a lot easier for your heart to do its job properly.

Other reasons could be the potassium in vinegar which some alternative practitioners claim can make the blood thinner.

Try taking a tablespoon diluted in water three times each day for a few weeks and see what happens.

High blood pressure is a very important health issue and could indicate a serious underlying problem, so talk to your doctor immediately if you are worried about this, and if you wish to make any dietary changes.

Bruises

Soak a cloth in some apple cider vinegar, together with some cold water. It acts as a compress, and draws the discoloration out of bruises.

Or for a traditional 'sage and vinegar' recipe:

Flatten some fresh sage leaves with a rolling pin. Simmer (don't boil) them in a pan, covered with vinegar, until the leaves soften. This should take no more than 5 minutes. Now fold the warm mix into a cloth and press against the bruise while still warm.

Burns

I don't need to tell you that a serious burn needs urgent attention from a medical professional, do I? However, if it's a minor burn...

Soak a piece of clean cloth in chilled vinegar and apply it to the affected area. Do this every 15 minutes until pain goes away.

Colds

Apple cider vinegar contains plenty of potassium which can help ease the formation of mucous, watery eyes, sinus and catarrh.

Mix a quarter of a cup of vinegar with a quarter of a cup of honey. Take a tablespoon six times each day. For a cough, try blending half a cup of vinegar with a half cup of water, adding in a teaspoon of cayenne pepper and four teaspoons of honey.

Take this whenever the cough gets bad.

Coughs

Here's one my mum used to swear by. Much to my horror. But it did work:

If you've got a cough, add 10 teaspoons of vinegar to a medium size pot of water and bring to the boil. Take it off the hob and put it on a safe surface. Grab a towel and drape it over your head. Now bend your head over the bowl and breathe in the steam.

Diabetes

Some researchers now believe that taking vinegar before a meal can help those who suffer from Type 2 diabetes. Carol Johnston, a professor of nutrition at Arizona State University, discovered this when she tried to develop the perfect menu for diabetics.

She found that taking two tablespoons of vinegar before a meal reduces the blood sugar 'spikes' you get after eating.

We all get these surges of glucose and insulin but for diabetics they are so powerful that they can cause problems like heart disease later in life. Luckily, the Type 2 diabetics who consumed vinegar saw this spike reduced by 25%. Even more excitingly it reduced these spikes by 50% for those people with signs of *future* diabetes.

In my view, the best way to have two spoons of vinegar before a meal would be to choose vinaigrette dressing on a tasty salad (See PART FIVE).

Disinfectant

Remember in PART TWO, how garlic soup was given to plague victims in the Middle Ages? Well, vinegar also has legendary status in the history of bubonic plague.

When it swept through France in 1721, the authorities ordered condemned prisoners to go out and bury the bodies. The legend has it that four robbers were caught looting possessions from abandoned homes in Toulouse. They were condemned to be hanged.

To save themselves they offered the people a deal. In return for their lives, they would give up the secret of how they remained immune to the plague. After revealing their mystery remedy, they were killed anyway.

Ah well, so it goes.

During my research, I've read many versions of this story. There are also many different versions of the remedy the robbers revealed before their deaths. It's still marketed today as 'Four Thieves Vinegar'. And while some websites I've seen claim it's a magical potion, I believe it's all down to the well-known antiseptic powers of vinegar.

Here's a way you can use Four Thieves Vinegar as an natural disinfectant:

> Place a small handful each of dried lavender, rosemary, sage, rue, garlic and mint in a large jar, and cover completely with organic apple cider vinegar. Cover tightly, put in the fridge and let it sit for six weeks. Strain away the garlic and herbs to leave a clear mixture.

Put this into a spray bottle and use on door handles, surfaces and infected areas of the home.

Food poisoning

When we get older, we sometimes produce less stomach acid. This means we can't fight enemy bacteria as easily, rendering us more likely to get infections from dodgy foods.

Vinegar's acetic acid can help fight the nasty bacteria in foods. One study I've read shows that 35% strength white vinegar can kill E. coli bacteria better than chlorine. So if you're on holiday abroad and you're worried about the food, get hold of some emergency vinegar.

> You can take a tablespoon of apple cider vinegar in warm water (with honey to taste) before each meal as a protective measure. Or in a case of food poisoning, take this mixture immediately.

Always stir well and let it cool a little before you drink it.

Fungal nail infection

This is one of those embarrassing subjects that people are loath to talk about. I mean, it's fine to tell your friends down the pub, "I keep getting these headaches". But you wouldn't interrupt a conversation to ask "Anyone know how to clear up nail fungus?" while slapping your bare foot on the table. That said, I actually have a few old university friends who probably would.

Fungal nail infections are caused by a fungus called onychomycosis, which is as difficult to say as it is embarrassing to have. The symptoms include thick and discoloured nails, brittle, misshapen nails, or pain in your toes.

There are many manmade prescription treatments for nail fungus, but most of the studies I've read reveal that they sometimes spark side effects like nausea, vomiting, dizziness, and fatigue.

So here's a natural alternative you should try before you resort to the expensive, artificial stuff. See if this doesn't clear it up quickly.

> Soak the affected nails for 15 minutes a day in a basin of warm water, with a cup of apple cider vinegar, and ten drops of lavender essential oil.

The vinegar restores the proper pH balance to the skin, toughening it up against infections, while the lavender has antimicrobial properties. Make sure you dry your feet thoroughly afterwards, as wet feet often trigger the problem in the first place. (For a true cautionary tale, see the section 'Athlete's Foot' in PART TWO!)

One more thing. If you're suffering this problem, don't wear pointed shoes that force your toes together (I realise this is very bad news for court jesters).

Even after you've fought off the infection, you'll need to keep your nails protected from a relapse. So get those clippers out and keep them neat and trim. Don't use the same nail trimmer or nail file that you use on healthy nails as you do on infected nails. Make sure you wear 100% cotton socks, and change your socks if they ever get damp from sweat or wet from splashing about in puddles like a child.

And take this final tip from a man who suffered a humiliating fungal foot infection in the prime of his mid-twenties: put on new socks every day, without fail, and try wearing flip flops around the house instead shoes or slippers.

Your loved ones may grimace, but fresh air will be your new best friend!

Haemorrhoids

One day, the young Ray Collins was ambling home from another boring day at school. Suddenly, the clouds parted, and a booming voice said to him: "Ray?"

"Yes?" squeaked the frightened child.

"You may not realise this, but a great destiny awaits you. One day your name shall be known by thousands of people across the kingdom."

The child tried to think what his destiny would be. Perhaps a great train robber, an actor, or even the first Welshman into space!

"That's right," boomed the voice in the clouds, "one day, you shall take it upon yourself to write to strangers about little-known ways they can deal with piles."

And lo, it came to pass. Here I am with a little vinegar trick that I was born to tell you.

Haemorrhoids are small, blood-filled swellings inside the anus. They itch and burn like hell. When it gets serious they can bleed. The first thing you must do is try and avoid constipation, one of the primary causes. Straining puts pressure on the veins, which can then swell, causing you untold agony.

Doctors then usually recommend a diet with more fibre and roughage – particularly green vegetables, fresh fruit, wholegrain cereals and at least 25 grams of bran each day. They'll also tell you to drink 8 to 10 glasses of fluid daily.

This is all good advice. But if you're suffering from piles, here's something else that can soothe the itching.

Soak a ball of cotton in a mix of vinegar diluted with water. Very, very gently, dab this on the affected area. This should shrink the blood vessels and ease the problem. Or take two teaspoonfuls of apple cider vinegar in a glass of water before each meal.

Headaches

Apple cider vinegar is a popular old wives remedy for headaches and migraines. Why it works, nobody truly knows. Some think that it's got something to do with the fact that, when you have a headache, your urine becomes more alkaline than usual. So perhaps vinegar's acid qualities rebalance the levels. The trick is to take it at the onset of your headache symptoms.

Mix 2 tablespoons of apple cider vinegar in 8oz of water, and take it two times a day. Add a tad more vinegar if it's a real pounder.

Another method is to try the steam therapy I describe in the section 'Coughs'.

Heartburn

Vinegar has long been a popular folk remedy for heartburn. While it might seem weird to counteract an acid flux reaction with a substance that's heavily acidic, it works for many people. Some believe, controversially, that because vinegar is acidic, your stomach slows or stops its acid production. The problem is that so few scientific tests have been carried out.

In my view, this is a huge shame. If vinegar was a patented drug that could make big pharmaceuticals an ocean of profit, they've have tested this a million times over. Of course, it isn't, so they don't. There's no money in it, so there's no available funding for research.

The result is that people like you miss out on a potentially cheap and effective cure for this everyday problem. Instead, you're encouraged to ignore all this folk-remedy nonsense and spend plenty of money at the chemist instead.

Give yourself the alternative option, even if it's merely to test the claims of millions of people through the decades. Try a vinegar remedy next time you get heartburn.

> When you've finished your meal, stir two tablespoons of apple cider vinegar into half a cup of pure apple juice or water and drink it down.

Make sure you're sensible with this. Try it once a day at most, and don't knock back increasing amounts of vinegar, as you could irritate your stomach lining.

Insomnia

In this weird and wonderful world, few things ever surprise me. Although when I discovered that Rolf Harris was a potential cure for insomnia, I was a little taken aback. No, it has nothing to do with his beard, or his songs, or his penchant for painting the Queen. His sleep remedy could be something to do with his musical passion.

Can you tell what it is yet?

Well, apparently, playing the didgeridoo could help alleviate sleep problems. Swiss researchers have that found using the instrument for 25 minutes a day helped people with sleep apnoea. Patients who had lessons reported less sleepiness during the day and their partners said there were fewer disturbances. It's all thanks to the breathing control involved in playing the instrument.

While this may be true, I don't think that the didgeridoo is an option for everyone. So try this simple vinegar remedy instead.

> Before you go to bed at night, mix two teaspoons of apple cider vinegar and two teaspoons of honey into a cup of hot water and drink steadily, but slowly.

This will only work if you follow a systematic and disciplined approach for getting over insomnia. So make sure you go to bed and wake up at the same time every day. This includes weekends. Always follow the same routine every night before going to sleep. For example, take a warm bath and then read for ten minutes.

Soon your mind will recognise these triggers and will start preparing for sleep.

If you're still awake after trying to fall asleep for half an hour, get up and read for a while, and drink another dose of the honey and vinegar mixture. Don't add too much water or you'll need to go for a wee within an hour.

An alternative is to add the vinegar to the honey without water and take a spoonful of the mixture, much like a cough medicine.

Joint Pain

Many nutritionists believe that apple cider vinegar could play role in fighting the causes of joint pain. According to many nutritionists, this is because vinegar contains natural enzymes that can help dissolve uric acid. These break down the calcium deposits lurking in your joints. At the same time, the vinegar builds up the minerals needed for a healthy bone structure.

If you want to benefit from the full power of apple cider vinegar, it should be unpasteurised, so these potent enzymes remain fully active.

But there's a problem. When it comes to supplying you with foods, it's not the nutritionists or doctors who dictate what you can and can't have – it's the marketing men. So, when it comes to apple cider vinegar, they take one look at it in its natural state and almost faint. All that colour, all those impurities... oh no, that just won't do.

Terrified of financial failure, they boil it to within an inch of its life, until it's clear and pretty and looks good on a shelf. This process kills all the enzymes and removes vital nutrients.

So if you want the most powerful anti-inflammatory nutrients fighting in your corner, make sure you use unpasteurised apple cider vinegar.

And here's another tip for you:

Although apple cider vinegar is good on its own, it's even BETTER if you take it with a powerful medicinal honey, like manuka honey, which I mentioned in PART ONE.

First off, the honey acts as a natural sweetener, so you don't have to hold your breath and think of England each time you swallow the vinegar. Secondly, manuka honey packs a few nifty health punches of its own – one of the main ones being its effectiveness as an anti-inflammatory.

So if you take a mixture of manuka honey with a good unpasteurised apple cider vinegar then BAM! Your joint pain won't know what's hit it.

Leg cramps

Muscle cramps are often caused by low potassium levels in your body. Take a teaspoon of vinegar at the onset of symptoms to recharge those potassium levels. You can also dab some vinegar on the cramped area use a soft cloth. The pain should subside fairly quickly.

> To prevent those painful leg cramps that come at night, drink a glass of water containing one tablespoon of vinegar with your evening meal.

Sore / smelly feet

Fill a washing up bowl with water and add half a cup of apple cider vinegar. Put your feet in the bowl, switch on the telly, and feel the soothing action. If you wash your feet with antiseptic soap first, this will also remove nasty foot odours.

Rosacea

This is nicknamed the 'curse of the Celts' by people in Ireland and Scotland. It begins as a red flush on the face and cheeks, nose, forehead, neck and chest. If you don't deal with it, over time your face will have permanent red lines from swollen and damaged veins

There was a case in Argentina of a 52-year old man who suffered Rosacea for 20 years, along with painful urination and other problems the doctors couldn't solve. He eventually found relief by taking vinegar and lemon every day.

I'd suggest a hot toddy consisting of the juice of half a lemon, a tablespoon of vinegar, two teaspoons of honey and hot water.

Stiff joints

In some cases, a shortage of potassium in your body can lead to stiff joints. Fill a bath with warm water. Add a small cup of apple cider vinegar. Get in and have a good soak.

Sunburn

Get some white distilled vinegar, put it in a spray bottle and leave in the fridge to get nice and cool. Now spray this on the burned area of skin. This should soothe and stop the blistering.

Tiredness

When you get stressed, your body releases lactic acid, which can lead to fatigue. Vinegar contains amino acids that can counter these lactic acids. Take a tablespoon of apple cider vinegar diluted in a little water every morning.

Upset stomach

Stir two teaspoons of apple cider vinegar into a cup of water and drink. This should take away the stomach upset. If you have diarrhoea, take a tablespoon of vinegar in a glass of water each hour until the problem goes away.

Or, on a more luxurious note, here's a wonderful way to ease the pain of irritable bowel syndrome:

> Fill a bath with warm water. Make sure it's not too deep. When you lie in it, the water should lap the sides of your stomach but your belly button should be above the water level. Add a cup of apple cider vinegar and Epsom salts. As an optional extra, try aromatic herbs like lavender or chamomile.
>
> Now relax in this bath for an hour with your legs over the side. Easy!

For more on stomach aches and pains, take a look at the section on honey, or search through the index at the back of this book.

CHAPTER THREE

How to choose and use your vinegar

Vinegar can be made from the fermentation of almost anything that contains natural sugars. As I explained in Chapter One, what happens is that yeast ferments the sugars into alcohol, and then bacteria turn that alcohol into vinegar.

This means that when you go to buy your vinegar, you're faced with a whole range of different types. Here are some of the main ones you'll see:

White distilled vinegar

This is made from ethanol and diluted with water. Not so good for cooking, this comes into its own when you want to try your hand at pickling. And it's possibly the best vinegar to use for cleaning the house. (See 'Allergies' for more details on this.)

Apple cider vinegar

Unsurprisingly, apple cider vinegar is made from apple cider. It is best for salads, dressings and marinades. It's also very good for general use around the home. Apple cider vinegar is highly acidic and can sometimes burn the throat if you don't dilute it. That said, it's good for pretty much every tip in this part of the book.

Red wine vinegar

Like apple cider vinegar, red wine vinegar is very versatile. It's popular in Mediterranean countries for using in sauces, salad dressings, marinades and as a pickling agent. As a rule, the better quality of the original wine the better the vinegar. When aged for a couple of years in wooden casks it gets a full, mellow and complex flavour.

White wine vinegar

Similarly to the red wine version, white wine vinegar comes from the fermentation of a selected blend of white wines. The result is a clear, pale, acidic vinegar.

Balsamic vinegar

This is produced in the Modena region of Italy from reduced grape juice aged in wooden casks. Dark brown in colour, it has a sweet 'n' sour flavour, making it an amazing dressing for salads and a brilliant marinade for steak. If you go for the genuine original Italian stuff, be prepared to shell out for it. Or you can try commercial versions from outside Modena.

Malt vinegar

This is the vinegar we Brits love to splash on our fish and chips. It is made from sprouted and fermented barley, then flavoured with woods like beech and birch. Some cheap versions are simply acetic acid with caramel colouring.

Mother of vinegar

This isn't actually a type of vinegar. Nor is it vinegar's real 'mother'. I don't think foodstuffs can have a mother. Although I've heard some people say that wine's mother is called Gladys. And that potatoes have an uncle called Alan.

Mother of vinegar is an unappealing, slimy residue found in unpasteurised vinegar. It's made up of acetic bacteria, the stuff responsible for turning alcohol into vinegar. When you pasteurise vinegar, you remove the 'mother'. Which is great for people who market and sell vinegar. Because they absolutely hate mother.

Mother means a far less attractive bottle of vinegar, and therefore a far less profitable bottle of vinegar. So they distil it to death. And sell it by the bucket-load. Hurrah!

However, when it comes to using apple cider vinegar as a natural health remedy, 'mother' is exactly what you want to see. Its murky presence means that the vinegar is brimming with active enzymes and essential nutrients.

As I said to my wife when convincing her to marry me: "In life, it's the ugly things that are the most good for you."

So for the maximum benefit from the tips in this part of the book, seek out some high quality, unpasteurised apple cider vinegar.

Twelve ways to use vinegar as your secret weapon in the kitchen

- Liven up beans and bean-based dishes. Add a dash of vinegar just in the last five minutes of boiling them. It will bring out the flavour.

- When braising meat in water, add some vinegar. It is said to tenderise the meat.

- To enhance the colour of vegetables, add vinegar to the water you're boiling them in.

- When you're boiling eggs, add vinegar to the water. This will make the eggs easier to peel afterward. It will also stop the egg white escaping from the shell while cooking.

- For poached eggs, before your put the eggs into the water, add a dash of vinegar. This helps keep them in one piece.

- Soak a cloth with vinegar, wrap your block of cheese in it and then keep it in the fridge in an airtight container. It should stay soft and mould free.

- Running out of ketchup but need an emergency dose to go with your chips? Add a little vinegar to the bottle and shake. You'll get that extra dash of ketchup without watering down the taste, as it contains vinegar anyway.

- To check if old baking soda is still okay to use, take a side plate and put a tablespoon of baking soda in the middle. Pour two tablespoons of vinegar on top. If it froths like mad, then it's okay. If it doesn't, then chuck it.

- When scaling fish rub it with vinegar first. This will make the job easier.

- Don't add salt to your pasta when you're cooking it. For a healthier option, add a tablespoon of vinegar to the pot. This will also stop the pasta sticking together.

- Or if you've just had a taste of your cooking and realised you've put in too much salt, it's vinegar to the rescue again. Add a spoonful of white distilled vinegar and a teaspoon of sugar. This should take away some of the saltiness.

- If, after chopping onions, your hands stink, rub them with vinegar to get rid of the smell.

The easiest dressing

One of the easiest ways to get a dose of vinegar into your diet is to make a vinaigrette.

The quickest option is to take one part vinegar and add it to three parts olive oil. Depending on your taste, you can use red wine vinegar, white wine vinegar or balsamic vinegar. The oil should be of really good quality to get the best result.

Once you've got the mix, add salt and pepper and whisk up, or shake in a jam jar.

In the Collins kitchen, I tend to experiment by adding honey, lemon, herbs, yoghurt, cream, or mustard to the dressing. You can make it as sweet and tasty as you like. I promise, once you've had a go, you'll never buy commercial dressings again. As long as you have vinegar and oil in your cupboards, you'll never be far from a tasty, healthy salad.

See PART FIVE for some great dressing recipes.

PART FOUR

CONFESSIONS OF A FAT MAN
The honey, garlic
and vinegar diet

CHAPTER ONE

How a fat man in Vietnam discovered the path to weight loss – without all the hunger, pain, and rabbit food

It was another hot day in coastal Vietnam. Cries and giggles drifted from the ramshackle market stalls at the foot of the Cham Towers, ancient religious monuments built between the 7th and 12th centuries AD.

As soon as we arrived at the tourist spot, children came running with beads, postcards, trinkets and bottled drinks for sale. Having been persuaded to buy a stack of rubbish postcards earlier that morning, I was reluctant to buy anything else.

"No, I already have some," I said, pulling the evidence out of my bag.

This made absolutely no difference. On the contrary, it indicated that *here was a man who bought postcards*. Therefore I was a man who could undoubtedly buy *more*. And if not, he would surely buy yet another coloured bangle for his wife. Or perhaps this, a luke-warm Coke, covered in dirt, and bottled sometime in 1989.

"No thanks," I pushed forwards. "Those look great, but no."

Then it happened. The curious thing. An incident which would, looking back on it, spark a chain of events that would end with me writing to you about honey, garlic and vinegar today. It was one of those turning points you get in life, where you see yourself as you really are for just one moment, and you're shocked into action.

What happened was this: one of the children put his hand on my stomach, a smile spreading across his face. Immediately, another did the same.

"Happy Buddha," he said, and walked away. As he did so, another child laughed. "Happy Buddha!" she said, and also patted my midriff.

"Why are you touching my stomach?" I said.

"For luck!" she cried. At which point, a bus load of German tourists pulled up behind us and they skipped away. I stared down at my belly in horror.

If you don't know already, the 'Happy Buddha' is the big fat bald character depicted in the popular statues. In the Far East his enormous, exposed belly is a symbol of happiness, good luck, and generosity.

While all this was fine, and I was glad to be of service, *'providing luck'* to the children of Vietnam, I was shocked. I'd never been a skinny man. Far from it. But to be seen as synonymous with the caricature of the Happy Buddha, well, it hadn't occurred to me that my weight issue had got so bad. Now I saw that my belly stuck out in front of me like a soft planet, or as if I were about to give birth to a dolphin.

How had this happened? *When* did this happen? *Why* hadn't I noticed it had gone this far?

Back at the hotel that evening I ordered a gin and tonic and brooded over my dietary behaviour.

A shocking realisation

In retrospect, my lifestyle had deteriorated badly.

Stressed and busy at my old office job. I had upped my calorie considerably and stopped doing any exercise at all. I had given up cigarettes a few months earlier. It felt like my metabolism was now so slow, I had turned into a giant, depressed slug.

My fingers, mouth and the depths of my soul needed some kind of replacement fix, and fast – now! Yes! Yes! *Give me FOOD!*

Constantly hungry, I travelled into work on the bus and bought sausage sandwiches from the canteen before I even got into the lift. I filled myself up with pasta salads and side-orders of sandwiches at lunch, followed by carrot cake, just to keep myself going. A woman with a sweet trolley came round in the afternoon, so I'd buy chocolate every day in rounds with my cubicle mate.

At nights I'd chomp my way through stuffed pasta in pesto, potato stews with side plates of white bread, or pizza. Before bed I'd often get a surge of ravenous hunger and eat slabs of cheese on crackers, or dunk huge chunks of pitta bread into dips.

In the morning I'd wake, almost crazed with hunger. If I happened to forgo my breakfast, I'd be so engrossed in fantasies about food at work, I'd spring, drooling from my desk at 11.59, so I could get the edge on the lunchtime queues.

For the first time ever, in that Vietnam hotel, absent-mindedly shovelling nuts into my mouth, I faced the truth: I was addicted to food. And I was no longer slightly overweight: I was unhealthily fat.

Worse, I was tired, unhappy, and very pessimistic that I could do anything about it.

Why starvation diets don't work

The problem was, the idea of dieting appalled and frightened me. Because, let's admit it, most dieters fail in their attempts. Or they succeed for a period of time, then the problem usually comes back worse than before.

A life of 'yo-yo' dieting can worse for your health than remaining overweight. Something the diet industry conveniently fails to tell you.

So when I got back to Britain I started researching everything I could find out about food. What went in it, what made you fat, what made you thin, and how you could kick the terrible food cravings and start a diet that really worked.

I quickly realised that wasn't about starving myself, giving up treats or munching through rabbit food. It was about changing my eating habits, and finding easy, natural ways to fight off food cravings. I didn't want to become thin, I wanted to become happy with myself. And I wanted to carry on enjoying food, but this time thinking about what was going into my body and making informed choices.

This was when I discovered the secret of successful dieting – and the amazing benefits of honey, garlic and vinegar.

The natural remedy that helps you slim

Soon my obsession changed from eating food to researching and writing about the health benefits of food. This was a far healthier habit. And when I gave up my office job, I was able to start my own weekly email newsletter, **The Good Life Letter**. This way I could share my experiences and discoveries with a growing army of readers.

By far the most popular topic I've uncovered is the *Honey Garlic and Vinegar* remedy I'm about to share with you. To give you an idea, I get emailed about it almost every month, with comments like this:

> *'I'm indebted to you for the weight loss from the honey, garlic and vinegar tablets. Weight had slipped on through the menopause. It wouldn't shift by the usual cutting-down methods and exercise, which had always worked in the past.*
>
> *Over a period of 18 months I spoke to my doctor, a dietician and a herbalist, read widely and tried some ideas from other companies. What I was looking for was a way-of-life diet so the weight would go off and stay off and I would be eating healthily as well.*

But it was the honey, garlic and vinegar tablets that actually worked and shifted much of the excess weight.

I have gone back to my original size in clothes, I feel very well and it's been a huge boost to my confidence. Furthermore the weight has stayed off, although I have not taken the tablets for a little while. I eat differently now and often include honey, garlic and cider vinegar in a meal".

On my website's shop, the supplement version of this remedy mentioned in the above email is the most popular product by far, with thousands of people choosing to buy it again and again. Yes, I've also come across sceptics who sneer at those who use honey, garlic and vinegar supplements to diet.

It's such a weird, controversial and popular idea, I thought to myself: "I'll annoy the hell out of the diet industry and the mainstream press, and stick the whole lot in a book!"

You see, you don't need to buy any supplements to make this work. You can get the benefits of honey, garlic and vinegar from the homemade recipe I'll show you in a moment. Also, this book is different, because I won't pretend for a second that it's a simple matter of eating these ingredients and magically watching the weight fall off.

The diet remedy I reveal in Chapter Two will ONLY work in combination with the important steps in Chapter Three. I advise you to read the whole of this part of the book before you try anything.

Okay?

Lovely, smashing, super. You win a speedboat.

CHAPTER TWO

The powerful combination that does you good

First off, let me show you how honey, garlic and vinegar are believed to aid weight loss on an individual basis.

Honey

When you eat refined sugar, you get an awful lot of calories and not much else. No minerals or vitamins. Honey is a far better replacement, in moderation, of course. Honey doesn't contain fat, cholesterol or salt. It's an unrefined natural sweetener packed with amino acids and minerals essential that help your body's metabolism tick over.

Many people use honey to kick start their metabolism in the morning. You simply squeeze lemon juice into a mug, add a spoon of honey, and drink it down warm. Or take a spoonful half an hour before breakfast.

Garlic

The most powerful active ingredient in garlic, allicin, has been shown to lower blood pressure, insulin and triglycerides in laboratory animals. This is according to The *American Journal of Hypertension*. The report also revealed that the animals who were given allicin didn't gain as much weight as those who weren't.

Garlic can also help your body break down lipids, which are the fat-soluble molecules in your body, including cholesterol.

Dr James Balch, author of *Ten Natural Remedies That Can Save Your Life* says, "Garlic also moves lipids from the tissue to the blood-stream for eventual removal. Garlic can dramatically reduce the bad consequences of a multitude of dietary sins."

A report in *The Lancet* suggested that you can even neutralise the effects of high fat foods by adding garlic to your diet. Researchers claimed that cholesterol levels dropped an average of 237.4 to 221.4 after volunteers took 50 grams of garlic and four ounces of butter.

Vinegar

Way back in 1958, Dr Deforrest Jarvis, a scientist from the University of Vermont, wrote a book called *Folk Medicine*. In this popular tome, he enthused about the effects of apple cider vinegar as a slimming aid.

From his observations, he surmised that weight loss using vinegar was slow and gradual, but effective. By taking two teaspoons of apple cider vinegar with water at every meal, he believed it would take a woman of average height, weighing approximately 95kilos, two years to slim down to 82 kilos.

Since then there hasn't been much research done, nor is there any money available for extensive research on natural foods like vinegar.

However, in October 2005, *The Daily Mail* reported on a new study that surprised a lot of people. Researchers from Sweden's Lund University found evidence that vinegar can work as an appetite suppressant. The reason was the vinegar helped reduce the amount of insulin your body produced after eating a carbohydrate meal.

This backs up the findings of Carol Johnston, a professor of nutrition at Arizona State University. As you'll have seen in PART THREE, she discovered that taking two tablespoons of vinegar before a meal reduces the blood sugar 'spikes' you get after eating.

To explain this quickly. When you eat a meal, your blood sugar levels rise, especially if you've eaten lots of sugary food, or food with a lot of refined carbohydrates in it (white rice, white flour, cake, white pasta).

To bring these levels down, your body produces a hormone called insulin. This causes a crash in your blood sugar. The crash causes a sudden feeling of hunger and emptiness.

It's this perpetual cycle of feeling stuffed, then empty, that can drive people to overeat, and reach for the wrong types of food. Because that peak of satisfaction you get from refined carbohydrates and sugars is actually very addictive.

Some experts believe that vinegar can help avoid that horrible crash, so you feel fuller more quickly, and for longer.

Honey, garlic and vinegar

As you've seen in this book, taken separately, honey, garlic and vinegar are all nutritious, healthy foods with a wide variety of health-giving properties. But many of my *Good Life Letter* readers have discovered that combining all three makes for a fantastic weight-loss aid.

Four international studies also claim that garlic and vinegar can help you lose weight:

- In China, 600 dieters were split into two groups. The groups who added garlic and vinegar to their diet lost an average of 10 pounds (4.5 kg) each week. This was double the amount lost by the group who didn't take a garlic and vinegar supplement.

- Dr. Hen Lee Tsno writing for in China's *Journal of Natural Medicines*, reported that patients given honey, garlic and vinegar before breakfast had a high reduction in high blood pressure and cholesterol in less than a week.

- A Russian study showed that after a month, dieters who used garlic and vinegar lost an average of 40 pounds. Those dieters who didn't, lost an average of just 22 pounds.

- Professor Carol S. Johnston a nutritionist at the Arizona State University East conducted a 4-week experiment to investigate the beneficial relationship between vinegar and diabetes. As an unexpected side effect she found that her test subjects lost weight! After taking two tablespoons of vinegar before each of two meals daily, the average weight loss over the four weeks was two pounds. Those that did not drink the vinegar showed no change.

Many naturopaths and researchers believe that when honey, garlic and vinegar are combined, something remarkable happens. They interact in your digestive system to increase the speed at which you lose weight and keep it off. Almost as if the trio bring the best out of each other. Like characters in an American 'buddy' film.

You can imagine the movie trailer for 'honey garlic and vinegar'.... *"When these crazy ingredients get together, nothing can stop them!"*

Many of my newsletter readers swear that, when used as part of a sensible eating programme for weight loss, these ingredients work more powerfully together than on their own. You can use honey, garlic and vinegar before and during meals to lower your appetite, reduce blood sugar spikes and encourage your body to store less fat. This remedy is completely natural and free of side-effects. And it's something you can easily make at home. Yes, that's right now – today! There's no excuse.

As long as you've got a jar of honey, some good quality vinegar and a bulb of garlic, you're ready to go. Here are a few ways to create your own honey, garlic and vinegar health tonic:

Take two cups of organic apple cider vinegar, eight garlic cloves, and a cup of honey. Blend in a mixer until the garlic is chopped. Store in the fridge. Then take a tablespoon of the mixture in a large glass of hot water every day.

Or here's another:

Add a tablespoon of honey, chopped garlic and two teaspoons of pure apple cider vinegar to warm water. Stir, let it steep for five minutes, then and drink. Make sure you've left the garlic out for 15 minutes without its peel before you chop it and use it.

Or here's a convenient way to create the above recipe in bulk, as recommended by of my newsletter readers:

> Something I used to do when making up my vinegar & honey. I would put 50ml of organic cider vinegar, add 50 ml of honey into a 500ml container, with minced garlic, then add hot water to the level. Then drink 50ml of the liquid each day.

These are all really good ways to get these three wonder foods into your diet. A more convenient alternative is to get hold of some pre-mixed bottles of unpasteurised apple cider vinegar and manuka honey. This way you've got an instant source of highly active ingredients you can drink directly, or use as a basis for dressings (see PART FIVE for some of my favourites),

You could also try out oral supplements that combine honey, garlic and vinegar in a pill that you take once a day.

For more details on both of these options, you can find free information on my website: **www.goodlifetter.co.uk**

CHAPTER THREE

The diet steps that could help honey, garlic and vinegar work for you

Before you try losing weight with honey garlic and vinegar, I need to make something very clear. You *must* have a serious eating programme in place before you pin your hopes on any medicine, remedy or supplement. Without a system to follow, and the willpower to follow that system, you're doomed to fail.

In the same way as nicotine patches won't wean a smoker off the fags unless they really want to quit, even the greatest miracle diet pill ever invented would fail for someone who hasn't targeted the source of their eating problem.

My advice is to analyse your eating habits. Write a food diary every day and tally up what you eat, when you eat, and how you feel afterwards. Talk to your doctor, too. Get as much information as you can about yourself before you start.

It was only after research that I found the method that worked for me.

What I discovered on my weight-loss journey

If, like me, you constantly crave snacks that give you instant gratification – like white bread, biscuits, bowls of white pasta, cakes, cereals – then think about trying a low GI diet. This means you choose to eat food with a low glycemic index.

As I explained in the previous chapter, foods with high GI act like sugar. They give you blissful high, until your blood sugar crashes and you're left ravenously hungry. Foods with low GI keep your blood sugar levels steady and you don't get trapped in a cycle of hunger.

The food industry makes a lot of money out of pushing high carbohydrate, high GI products. They repackage them as 'low fat' and encourage you to diet by munching bowls of cereal in the morning. These include bowls of snack pasta for lunch, and lots of 'low fat' spreads, crisps, and other modified foods.

The problem is that the diet industry has been singing this tune since the '70s. The majority of people who have dieted have typically cut out red and fatty meats, replacing them with lots of chicken, fish, carbohydrates and vegetables. Millions – nay, *billions* – of people have been on these diets for decades.

And yet we're getting *fatter*.

According to a government report in 2007, 60% of UK men, 50% of women and a quarter of all children could be clinically obese by 2050.

It's never the processed high-carb products which fill the super-market shelves that get the blame for all this. Instead, it's all blamed on fat and meat.

It can get ridiculous. Even high-brow newspapers and television programmes tow the food industry line on this. Let me give you an example to show you what I mean. Last year, while watching Channel 4 News, I was gobsmacked to see Jon Snow announce: 'Meat causes cancer: it's official.'

A big photo of bacon flashed onto the screen with a red line through it, as if it was a paedophile, or Hitler.

The story was that The World Cancer Research Fund (WCRF) had released a report, based on studies dating back to the 1960s. They've been looking at reasons for, and solutions to, the growing global obesity crisis. Among the many conclusions in the report, was that scientists believe there is 'convincing' evidence that red meat and processed meats such as ham, bacon, salami and sausages increase the risk of colorectal cancer, and this was linked to obesity.

So the upshot is that meat is the reason we're getting fatter and more prone to cancer. But do you think the Channel 4 report concentrated on all the *other* powerful health issues?

Did they talk about all the contributing factors to obesity and cancer? You know, things like lack of exercise, environmental toxins, sugary foods, booze consumption and general over-consumption, too many refined carbohydrates, poor nutritional education, additives and other chemicals in ready meals, or fast food advertising?

No. It was all about, "DANGER! Your sausage means DEATH! Run for the hills!"

Why you should look past the scaremongering

While I assume there's meat involved in gaining weight, I'd put a wager on the fact that it also involves eating lots of bread, pasta, dairy, sugar, cakes, chocolate and soft drinks. Also, I'd also take a look at the basic cause of all weight gain: *consuming more than your body can burn* as fuel.

Of course, as soon as anyone suggests this, you get the naysayers in the press crying out: "Ah, you're another evil-doer, peddling these low-carb crash diets that mean you have to eat cheese, cream and steak ALL DAY FOREVER".

This is not true. Yes, lots of the advertising for these low-GI diets tries to hook you with promises of eating unhealthy food *and* losing weight. These make it more dramatic and appealing. You may have seen the ads that show you can guzzle lots of surf-n-turf meals and cream. Why? I suppose most people react to big, controversial promises that make them think they can eat rubbish and still be as thin as Kate Moss.

Remember, this is *advertising*. The peddlers of the diet programmes are trying to reach as many desperate people as possible with a big promise.

I'll admit this isn't an ideal situation, but the big players who advertise their processed foods on television are *doing the same thing*.

The truth you don't hear often is that these diets merely have a two-week period where, yes, you cut out a lot of food groups and lose a lot of weight quite quickly. This is so you kick the cravings, reset your eating habits, and go through cold turkey. It's also to motivate you by seeing *instant* success.

You're not expected to stay on these for any unhealthy length of time. Or lose the same amounts of weight thereafter. Over the following stages of all decent diets, you will introduce fruits and juice, brown rice, brown bread, brown pasta and all the vegetable groups. Contrary to most people's knowledge, a classic low-GI diet would see you eating at least one carb (like potatoes or brown bread) per day.

It's the refined carbohydrates that you need to cut down on. The stuff that acts like sugar, giving you the highs and crashing lows. White bread, white rice, biscuits, cakes, chips, pizza dough for example.

And no, the dinners are not all dangerously high fat. Low GI meals include things like grilled chicken with a large salad. Or grilled fish with green beans or leeks. Fresh tomato soup. Garlic mussels with brown bread.

So what I suggest is that you find a balanced diet that involves less refined sugar, fewer processed foods and fatty snacks. Meanwhile, eat more nuts, fruits, grilled meat and vegetables.

Hardly an unsustainable or dangerous diet is it?

Why rules matter

That said, this book is not supposed to lecture you or tell you what to do. Different methods work for different people, and it's up to you what kind of diet you pick.

My only recommendation is that you do follow a set of rules, as they will keep you focused and allow you to measure your intake carefully each day, setting achievable goals. As with giving up smoking, kicking a food addiction requires discipline.

Having rules also allow you to *relax* these rules as time goes on, so that you can give yourself rewards and treats.

Give it a go. You'll find that merely the act of *observing what you eat* every day will change your habits and help you lose weight. This is because it makes you aware of exactly what's going into your mouth, and what effect it has.

How it worked for me

To help you get started, here's the rough eating plan I followed, and still follow to a large extent. It got me over my addiction to sugar and refined carbs, and helped me gradually lose over a stone in less than six months. Weight that I have since kept off.

Okay, so my belly still bulges a bit. Yes, I could be accused of being "cuddly" by polite strangers. But it no longer looks like Jupiter is trying to burst out of my stomach, or that a witch's curse has given me 11 chins. I like to believe that on a future visit to Vietnam I won't be mistaken for the Happy Buddha.

Please note that at no point did I go hungry or miss out on vegetables, carbohydrates or the tasty food I loved. All it took was some concentration, time and effort to make sure I simply didn't reach for the easiest option, shove a pile of cheese between two slices of white bread, grab a bag of crisps and waddle out the door!

Breakfast

TIP: Get up fifteen minutes earlier, and take longer over breakfast. Half an hour before you eat, drink a mug of manuka honey and lemon tea with a teaspoon of apple cider vinegar stirred in. Or try one of the smoothies from PART FIVE.

Try a brisk walk after breakfast, either to work, to the bus stop, or round the garden. This will get your metabolism up and running for the day.

My breakfast choices:

• Scrambled eggs and smoked mackerel

• Fruit, yoghurt and honey (see the Honey Yoghurt Breakfast recipes in PART FIVE).

• Boiled eggs and 100% wholegrain bread.

To drink:

• Freshly squeezed juice. To get the maximum vitamin C, try grapefruit or lemon juice or kiwi fruit. A kiwi fruit contains five times the amount of vitamin C than an orange. Squeeze the juice freshly yourself and drink it right away. It loses vitamins almost instantly.

• Coffee. I'm a fan of coffee, and dislike the general bad press it gets. Years ago it was perceived to be an evil only equal to nicotine. Coffee stood accused of causing headaches, mood swings, bad breath, heart palpitations and stress.

  Now a growing number of people believe that the caffeine in coffee could lower your risk of diabetes and Parkinson's disease. It actually stimulates your brain and can lift your mood in the morning. Just keep it to a cup of good filter coffee each morning.

Lunch

TIP: Eat soup as your regular lunch. It tricks your stomach into feeling fuller more quickly.

My choices were:

• Salad with manuka honey, garlic and vinegar dressing. If you thought lettuce was useless and weedy, think again. Lettuce is the Clark Kent of the vegetable world. It may seem weak and nerdy, but it contains high levels of iron and magnesium, two substances that give your liver a real boost. They're also excellent diuretics, and wash away fatty cells like nobody's business.

• Any kind of soup really, as long as it's fresh, using natural ingredients. Homemade is best, of course.

• If you didn't have oily fish for breakfast, now is the time to try the mackerel recipe revealed in PART FIVE.

Dinner

TIP: Eat your evening meal earlier. You will burn more calories while you're up and active than during sleep. Try and include soy beans in a meal at least twice a week. They contain a substance called lecithin (there's a clue in the name). It helps form a shield around your cells so that fat can't wriggle in and plump them up.

My choices were:

• Grilled chicken with asparagus - this vegetable contains asparagines; an alkaloid that stimulates the kidneys and improves circulation. It also contains a chemical that breaks up oxalic acid - a type of natural glue that makes fat stick to you.

- Fish with plenty of green vegetables or salad.

- Lean red meat with salad or roasted root vegetables.

- Vegetable stew including lentils and beans.

- Chili con carne with brown rice.

To drink:

- Honey, garlic and vinegar drink (recipes in Chapter Two of this part of the book). Take this half an hour before you eat.

- Mineral water – drinking water helps your stomach believe that it's full.

- Red wine – wine contains 'flavonoids', antioxidants which keep cholesterol from damaging your artery walls. Many scientists now believe that a glass of red wine a day could help keep heart disease at bay.

- Don't like red wine? Then get hold of some purple grape juice. If you have a juicer, even better, as you will ensure you get all those flavonoids locked inside a fresh grape's skin.

Snacks

TIP: Make a huge fruit salad to pick at. Sometimes the appeal of snacking is simply the fact it's no bother. So make a big bowl of fresh fruit salad, and stick it in the fridge - right at the front where you'll see it immediately. When you come over all zombie-like with food cravings, and open the door muttering 'Yeeees master', you can simply grab the fruit salad and munch away.

Another of my top tips is to keep bags of nuts handy at all times. Here are my favourites:

- Pistachios – according to a report in the *Journal of the American College of Nutrition* they can produce a 10 point drop in your triglycerides and a 16 point decline in your levels of LDL cholesterol. That's the 'bad cholesterol' so everyone say "boooo".

- Walnuts – they contain omega 3s which may help ward off depression and heart attack, according to Harvard research.

- Brazil nuts – they contain selenium, a mineral linked to prostrate cancer protection, according to scientists at the University of Arizona.

- Pecans – these have the most antioxidants of any nut. Used as part of a healthy diet, they could help reduce your risk of cancer, heart disease and Alzheimer's disease.

- Hazelnuts - a handful daily could boost your levels of HDL cholesterol (the 'good' cholesterol, everyone cheer "hussah!") by 12%, according to a study published in the *European Journal of Clinical Nutrition*.

If you don't like nuts, consider 'soy nuts'. These are dried and roasted soybeans. They have many of the same health benefits as nuts, but aren't officially nuts. You should also track down some flax seeds, pumpkin seeds or sunflower seeds.

While I'm on the subject, don't be fooled by the many so-called 'health bars' and cereals on the market. They may contain nuts, but they do nothing for you.

Energy bars pretend to be health foods simply by adding some fibre. Sugary cereals boast that they're good for you because they've added some vitamins. But these are no substitute for the real thing - whole foods with natural sugars, vitamins and fibre.

That said, this eating plan isn't about depriving yourself of the good stuff. So allow yourself treats.

My weapons of choice?

• Dark chocolate - this has many benefits. It is rich in antioxidants that help your blood vessels work properly. Some researchers now believe that a few squares of dark chocolate a day may help to keep dementia at bay by improving the blood supply to your brain. Chocolate also contains phenylethylamine (PEA). Apparently PEA releases the same feel good hormones circulated after lovemaking.

Please note the word 'after'. It is not, as my wife claims, a replacement for the real thing.

• Cheese – I could never, EVER go without cheese. It's my feel-good food. So I regularly enjoy chunks of feta in my salad, parmesan on my vegetables. At least once every couple of days I eat some mature tangy cheddar and apple. Delicious.

By following a similar plan to mine, and by using the honey, garlic and vinegar recipes as a way to minimise your cravings, you should start to lose weight fairly quickly. But it's not just what you eat that's important, it's how you eat.

How your eyes can trick you into eating less

Everybody knows that to get slim you have to watch the amount you eat. Sounds obvious, doesn't it?

But do you really know how much you are eating?

A scientist in the US has discovered that people are terrible at estimating the actual amount they eat during any given meal. Dr Brian Wansink, director of the 'Food and Brand Lab' at the University of Illinois, believes that the size of our plates and glasses may be linked to weight gain.

He has spent his career studying how the size of our plates, glasses and food packaging influences our eating habits. His conclusion is that the bigger your plate, the fatter and rounder your glass, the more you will eat and drink.

For example, people who gulp from short, fat glasses drink will twice as much as those who use tall, slender glasses – even when the glasses hold the same volume.

Warsink's view is that it's your eyes that calculate how much you are eating. They decide you are full or not, much more so than your stomach. He has backed this up with dozens of odd experiments.

Here are my favourites:

- In one experiment, Wansink's researchers rigged up some self-filling soup bowls and normal bowls. They found that those who couldn't see the levels of their soup going down ate 40% more than those who ate from normal bowls.

- In another, they asked 48 bartenders to pour a gin and tonic into either a tall glass or a short, wide tumbler. They were supposed to pour a shot, but they didn't have a shot glass to measure with. The bartenders poured an average of 26 percent more alcohol into the wide tumbler than the tall glass.

- In a Chicago cinema, they randomly gave people medium or large buckets of popcorn. Those with big buckets ate roughly 50% more than those with medium. But when asked to estimate how many ounces or calories they had eaten, there was no difference between what the two groups reported.

Who said science wasn't fun?

The great thing about this revelation is that you can get slimmer simply by eating the same food, but less of it. With a few nifty optical illusions you can feel more satisfied during and after each meal.

My tip? Go out today and buy smaller plates and thinner glasses. Use these for all your meals. When it comes to salads and fruit, use larger bowls so that you eat more of the healthy stuff. If you want to enjoy a treat, put them into small bowls.

Now it's up to you

All the above strategies work well for me. But it's up to you to analyse your own food habits and find that perfect eating plan for you. Not a crash diet or fad you go though for a month or two. Something you can sustain for the rest of your life.

Follow some palatable rules and, instead of falling on and off the wagon, you should be able to adjust your eating habits permanently. Hopefully you will find this far easier with the help of honey, garlic and vinegar, undoubtedly three of nature's miracles.

PART FIVE

THE CHEF'S HEALTH KICK:
14 delicious honey, garlic and vinegar recipes

About these recipes

While I'm often seen brandishing a colander, whisking eggs and plunging my arm into bald chickens, I'm not a chef. The fact that I like to wear a tall white hat around the house and talk endlessly about "drizzling" is beside the point.

However, I do like collecting and adapting recipes that incorporate the natural wonders of honey, garlic and vinegar. I mean, what's the point of writing about these foods without trying your hand at eating them properly?

Even so, I felt that for this part of the book I'd ask for some expert help. Yes, I could pass on some of Collins' culinary tips to you. But I'm very aware that many cooking processes change the chemistry of honey and vinegar.

If you're too cavalier about cooking with these ingredients, you'll remove many of the health benefits before you even lift your knife and fork.

So I contacted Sally Fenn, a nutritionist who works with a company called Green Bay Harvest (http://www.greenbayharvest.co.uk/productsSweetRemedies.asp). They specialise in producing top notch Manuka Honey (see PART ONE for details). They also create super-healthy mixtures of apple cider vinegar and honey for the international market.

Between us, we come up with a range of simple recipes that provide the benefits of honey, garlic and vinegar.

Not to spoil your fun, I've also included a few that, because of the cooking process, don't necessarily keep all the goodness described in this book – but taste damned good anyway. I'll indicate whenever this has happened.

This isn't a cook book, so please don't expect culinary genius. I'll leave that to the Jamie Olivers and Gordon Ramsays of this world. But I hope you'll discover some really quick and tasty ways to get all the health benefits of this book, without feeling that you're throwing medicine down your throat.

After all, these ancient ingredients are to be enjoyed and revered. They're nature's miracle, not a painful chore! These recipes should give you ideas about how you can start introducing honey, garlic and vinegar – in healthy amounts – into your diet. They're here for you to adapt to your tastes and needs.

On a final note, I've kept to one recipe per page so you can flatten out my book, and easily peer at the instructions while you cook. If you're a messy type and the pages get spattered in gunk, then I highly recommend buying another copy of *The Honey Garlic and Vinegar Miracle*.

I suggest you keep your second copy pristine in a glass box. Seal it up. Leave a tiny little hammer beside it in case of emergencies. When you're in dire need of some exciting natural remedies and recipes, you'll know exactly what to do.

Enjoy.

The recipes

Fennel, orange and chicken salad

This simple recipe uses a healthy mixture of apple cider vinegar and honey for a delicious, quick lunch.

For the salad:

- 1 fennel bulb, finely sliced
- 250g cooked chicken, roughly shredded
- 2 oranges, peeled and segmented
- Small handfuls of fresh parsley and mint

For the dressing:

- 1 ½ tbsp olive oil, 1 ½ tbsp flax oil
- 1 tbsp apple cider vinegar or apple cider vinegar with active manuka honey
- Pinch of flaky sea salt
- Freshly ground black pepper

Directions:

- First, combine the salad ingredients in a bowl.
- Then whisk up the dressing – or place everything in a sealed jar and shake vigorously
- Now pour over the salad.

Serves two.

Mackerel, rocket and new potato salad

Here you not only get the benefits of the honey and vinegar dressing, you'll get a boost of omega 43 fatty acids from mackerel, a fantastic oily fish.

For the salad:

- 2 fillets cooked mackerel, smoked or fresh
- 300g new potatoes, boiled in their skins
- 2-3 finely chopped spring onions
- 2 handfuls rocket leaves

For the dressing

- 1 ½ tbsp olive oil, 1 ½ tbsp flax oil
- 1 tbsp apple cider vinegar or apple cider vinegar with active manuka honey
- Pinch of flaky sea salt
- Freshly ground black pepper

Directions:

- Place the new potatoes and spring onions in a bowl
- Make the dressing and pour over the potatoes and onions
- Break the fish into large chunks, add to the mix, then tip the salad onto rocket leaves on a large plate.

Serves two.

Beetroot, goats cheese and Puy lentil salad

This one is fantastic because as well as apple cider vinegar, this is an easy way to get some beetroot into your diet. Known as 'the vitality plant', beetroot is rich in vitamins and minerals like iron and magnesium. In the past it was known to help treat anaemia and boost the immune system.

For the dish:

- 8 cooked beetroot
- 1-2 small goat cheeses – or chevre is fine
- 2tbsp fresh mint, chopped
- 1 red onion, thinly sliced
- 300g puy lentils, cooked
- 2tbsp apple cider vinegar
- 2 tbsp flax oil
- Grated zest ½ orange
- Chunky sea salt

Directions:

- Combine oil, vinegar, salt and orange zest. Gently combine remaining ingredients and dress.

Tomato salad dressing

Here's an easy dressing that combines vinegar and garlic to great effect. You could also add a touch of honey to this to get the entire trio in one tasty dish!

- 1 handful cherry tomatoes, chopped small
- ½ clove garlic, crushed
- 2 tbsp olive oil, 2 tbsp flax oil
- 2 tbsp apple cider vinegar
- 1 handful basil, chopped
- Pinch chilli powder, if desired

Directions:

- Combine the ingredients and pour over rice, pasta or green salads.

Easy Honey and Mustard dressing

If you want decent shot of honey but don't want to simply spoon it into your mouth, then this is the quickest and easiest way to add it to almost any meal.

Ingredients:

- A tsp of cream or crème fraich
- A tsp of dijon mustard
- A tsp of manuka honey
- 1 tbsp of white wine vinegar
- 3 tbsp of olive oil

Directions:

- Whisk together the ingredients or shake them up in a jar.

Even EASIER apple cider dressing

If you want to enjoy the benefits of vinegar every day, simply create a big jar of this...

Ingredients:

- 3 tbsp apple cider vinegar
- 9 tbs extra virgin olive oil
- Salt
- Pepper

Directions:

Mix the ingredients, adding more oil if you like, and seasoning according to taste. If you'd like to add extras, try some honey, herbs and crème fraich.

Honey, Garlic and Vinegar dressing

For the mother of all dressings, and not for the faint hearted, try this combination of all 3 ingredients in this book

Ingredients:

- 1 clove of roasted garlic (cook in the skin and then squeeze out the soft centre, which can be easily mixed)
- 1 tbsp of manuka honey
- 2 tbsp of cider vinegar
- 4 tbsp of olive oil
- 1 tbsp crème fraich
- Sea salt
- Black Pepper

Directions:

- Get these ingredients well-blended, shaken and mixed. This one is a bit of a Collins concoction so as you make it, alter the amounts and seasoning to suit your taste. Use a salad leaf to test the mix as you go.

Roasted roots salad

Here's another super-healthy dish that involves garlic and apple cider vinegar. Again, you can opt to add some manuka honey to the dressing if you'd like it sweeter, or simply need a honey boost!

Ingredients:

- 7 tbsp olive oil
- 4 large carrots, trimmed, scrubbed and quartered lengthways
- 4 large parsnips, trimmed, scrubbed and quartered lengthways
- 1 large red onion, peeled and cut in thin wedges
- Sprigs of thyme
- 1 head garlic, broken into cloves
- 2 large handfuls salad leaves, such as endive, rocket etc
- 1 handful fresh parsley, chopped
- 1 ½ tbsp apple cider vinegar

Directions:

- Heat oven to 220 C, gas mark 7.
- Pour 2 tbsp oil into a roasting dish on the hob and heat.
- Add the carrots and parsnips and cook for 5 minutes
- Add the onions and cook for another 5 minutes, stirring.
- Add the herbs and garlic, pour over 2 tbsp oil, season and roast for 30 minutes, turning once.
- Leave to cool for 10 minutes.
- Add 3tbsp of olive oil to 1 ½ tbsp apple cider vinegar (with a touch of honey if you'd like it sweeter) and tip onto the leaves and parsley.

Honey, Garlic and Vinegar Chicken Wings

This is another recipe with all three of our star performers, but this one is about flavour more than the health benefits, as cooking them all up like this will alter the enzymes and their actions. That said, it's finger lickin' tasty.

Ingredients:

- Approximately 15 chicken wings
- ¼ cup liquid honey
- 2 minced garlic cloves
- 1 tbsp apple cider vinegar
- ½ cup hoisin sauce
- ¼ cup soy sauce
- 1 tbsp chicken stock

Directions:

- Mix the hoisin sauce, soy sauce, honey, stock, cider vinegar and garlic.
- Add wings to the marinade, cover and refrigerate for 4 hours, turning occasionally.
- Take it out of the fridge, remove the wings, and put the marinade to one side.
- Place the wings on a greased baking tray, and cover with half the marinade.
- Back at 400 F for 20 minutes.
- Turn over the wings and brush with rest of the marinade
- Cook for another 20 minutes or until the juices run clear
- Now place under the grill for a minute per side to get the wings crispy.

Orange, Carrot and Honey Juice

I advise anybody who wants to enjoy a healthy life to get a juicer. This way you can create wonderful tasty juices into which you can add almost any ingredient you like. Here's an example:

Ingredients:

- 3 whole carrots
- 1 whole orange
- 1 tbsp honey

Directions:

- Juice the carrots and orange, then stir in runny honey (heat the honey gently in the jar, placed inside a pot of simmering water to get the right consistency)
- Stir vigorously, add ice and drink.

Honey Milk Shake

This is so easy, so tasty, and so what if the ice cream isn't such a healthy ingredient. A bit of what you fancy does you good. Especially if it contains honey!

For the shake:

- 43g Vanilla ice cream
- 1 tbsp of honey
- 1 cup of milk

Directions:

- Chuck it all in a blender and whizz it around until smooth. If your honey is a little too well set, place the jar in a pot of simmering water until it starts to go runny, then remove and it should blend nicely into the milkshake.

Honey Yoghurt Breakfast

For something as simple as the idea on the previous page, but far healthier, you could try this...

Ingredients:

- Your favourite natural yoghurt
- As many spoonfuls of honey as you like
- Chopped banana
- Chopped nuts of your choice.

Directions:

- Mix the lot and wolf it down. This has to my favourite breakfast of all time.

Garlic and Vinegar Dip

Here's a nice way to enjoy garlic and vinegar. You can use this as a dip for raw vegetables or a topping for baked potato. Or slap a dollop of this next to a juicy steak. Anything you like, really.

Ingredients:

- 1 crushed garlic clove
- ½ cup of plain yoghurt
- ½ cup mayonnaise
- 1 tbsp apple cider vinegar
- Salt
- Black pepper

Directions:

- Simply mix up the ingredients and enjoy!

Whole Baked Sea Bass with Garlic

Here's one that's easy to prepare, and is my ultimate favourite Saturday lunch. If you've got a few quid spare for a large, line caught wild sea bass, then you can't beat this. A massive fish, stuffed with good stuff.

Ingredients:

- One large, whole sea bass, gutted and scaled (ask your fishmonger to do this for you if you're squeamish. I like them to keep the head on, too).
- 2 tbsps white wine vinegar
- 1 lemon, sliced
- 2 whole cloves of garlic + 1 chopped clove of garlic
- 1 small red or yellow pepper
- 1 onion cut into thin rings
- Handful chopped parsley
- Sprig of rosemary
- Salt
- Pepper
- Olive oil

Directions:

- Brush both sides of the fish with oil then season with salt and pepper.
- Stuff the inside of the fish with two small whole cloves of garlic, skin off, and the sprig of rosemary.
- Place the fish in a foil parcel or baking parchment, anything to seal it as it cooks.
- Add the vinegar.
- Sprinkle with parsley and the chopped garlic

- Cut the pepper into thin strips and lay alongside the fish
- Cover the fish in the strips or rings of onion
- Add slices of lemon
- Seal the parcel and cook in the oven at 220 degrees for 15 – 25 minutes depending on the size of the fish.
- To check it's cooked, open the parcel and tug at the flesh with a fork, if the skin breaks and the flesh flakes away easily, you're ready to go.

Serve with a side salad to two hungry people.

Afterword

I hope you've enjoyed reading this book as much as I've enjoyed writing it. My vision is for a Britain where people can freely discuss alternative health remedies and have some fun on their quest to live happier lives.

Imagine a world where we clean our homes without toxins... save money on expensive remedies by making our own superior versions... and enjoy the bounty nature has provided us... where we can access knowledge of all kinds... and make our own decisions about how we look after our minds and bodies.

Or, alternatively, imagine a book like this in a big pile of other natural health books. Banned, ignored, on fire.

I know which world I'd prefer to live in.

If you'd like to hear more of my recipes, tips, rants and raves, you're more than welcome to visit my website, **The Good Life Letter**. You'll be able to browse through four years worth of my articles for free. Or sign up for the twice-weekly email newsletter and get it all delivered directly to your inbox.

Go to www.goodlifeletter.co.uk

Index

<u>Notes</u>

Notes

<u>Notes</u>

Notes

<u>Notes</u>

<u>Notes</u>

<u>Notes</u>

<u>Notes</u>

Notes

Praise for *The Lemon Book,* by Ray Collins

"I keep reading your Lemon Book over and over as there is so much good info.... Everything is written in laymans language and is a pleasure to read."
Tom Dooley, Hants

"There are lots of good and useful tips written and presented in a pleasant, citrusy and zestful way. Very good little book, I only wish I'd thought of writing it!"
John McLelland

"My skin will be rejuvenated, my house pristine and my clothes stainless – what more can a girl ask!! Thanks and keep up the good work."
Pauline (Uphill)

"As a result of buying the Lemon Book I am now a 'Lemon' convert! I found it easy to read, understand & very practical. I look forward to the next one!"
Finola

"So much good natural advice. Looking forward to the next book.
G Land

"I cannot remember the last time I have enjoyed reading such a brilliant book, it has brought back laughter and smiles. Thank you so much.
Sue Mould

"My father has just given me your Lemon Book. I love it and really enjoy your writing style. I have just had a look at your web site and am looking forward to further visits over the next few weeks. Its packed with such great ideas."
Joanna Russell

"Having purchased your lemon book I was pleased and very surprised (old cynic that I am) to find that the tip of adding lemon juice to light washes to bring the white, works so very well. The timely reminder of using a piece of the lemon peel in the waste disposal to stop it from becoming smelly was most appreciated too – a sweet smelling waste disposal has returned to this household. Sincere thanks for all that research."
Marianne – London

"There is so much information that is new to me and I will enjoy trying them out."
Linda Watt"

"Excellent reading. I learned quite a few tips... and I like lemons too."
Bernard

Copies are available now at
www.lemonbook.co.uk